CLINIC LAUNCH —SECRETS—

A HEALTHCARE PROFESSIONAL'S PLAYBOOK FOR BOOSTING INCOME AND AUTONOMY THROUGH PRACTICE OWNERSHIP

JASON A. DUPRAT

CLINIC LAUNCH SECRETS

A Healthcare Professional's Playbook for Boosting Income and Autonomy through Practice Ownership

For permission requests, speaking inquiries, podcast interviews, and bulk order purchase options, email support@jasonduprat.com.

Book Design by Transcendent Publishing | transcendentpublishing.com
Editing by Lori Lynn Enterprises
JASONDUPRAT.com

ISBN: 979-8-9878728-0-2

Printed in the United States of America.

WHAT OTHERS HAVE SAID

"Making the decision to leave certainty for uncertainty is difficult for most, especially if you have worked as hard as you have to hold a career in the healthcare industry. If anyone knows exactly what that is like, it's Jason Duprat. He's decoded the exact process that healthcare workers can use to leverage their skill and experience in an entrepreneurial venture that allows them to achieve the level of fulfillment they desire along with financial and time freedom that they never thought would be possible. This book will teach you that process. I highly recommend it."

—Travis Chappel,
Founder of Guestio, Host of *Travis Makes Friends*

"I don't give endorsements lightly, but I would highly recommend that anything Jason is saying, clinic owners should pay attention to. I only wish I had met Jason sooner. Who knows where I would be at? I fully believe what Jason has taught me will take my 7-figure clinic to an 8-figure clinic most likely in the next 5 years. Remember you can't go backward in time, but you can fast-forward with mentorship. With Jason's courses, he will not only educate you but also help with implementation. Information without implementation is not very helpful. I like the quote from Derek Sivers: 'If more information was the answer, then we'd all be billionaires with perfect abs.'"

—Dr. Eric Ehle,
DO, Medical Director of Well Life Family Medicine

"You absolutely do not have to remain in a corporate healthcare setting to be a successful healthcare professional. There are so many business opportunities out there. This book will address many common challenges faced when starting a clinic, and the content contained here will help you learn how to overcome them. Since you are reading this book, you're already on the right path. I'm excited for you and confident that this book will help streamline your path to success. I am sure you will enjoy it."

—Paul Colligan,
DNP, APRN, CRNA, PHN

TABLE OF CONTENTS

Dedication vii

Foreword. ix

Section I — Making the "Big" Decision 1

   1. The Wake-Up Call 3

   2. The Most Gratifying Benefits of Self-Pay Clinics . . . 17

   3. Mindset: The "Holy Grail". 41

Section II — Business Planning: Setting the Pace
to Become a Healthcare Boss 71

   4. Turning Your Dream into a Vision,
      Then into Your Reality 73

   5. Market Research and Analysis 81

   6. Financial Planning: Know Your Numbers. 89

   7. Designing Your Practice for Jaw-Dropping Success . . 113

Section III — Insanely Valuable Need-to-Knows 131

   8. Regulatory and Legal Planning: Avoiding the
      Pitfalls That Could Set You Back 133

9. Incorporation: The "Why" and the "How" 149

10. Insurance: Protecting Yourself from the Unknown . . 159

Section IV — Getting Started: Excited? You Should Be!   171

11. Selecting the Perfect Office Space on a Budget 173

12. Crack the Code: Understanding Commercial Leases . 183

13. Supplies and Equipment: Crucial Details
    You Need to Know. 189

14. Human Resources: Your Boom or Doom 197

**Section V — Next Steps: Roll Up Your Sleeves and
    Get Ready to Crush It 209**

15. Streamlining: How to Stand Out and Make Your
    Competitors Irrelevant 211

16. The Explosive Power of Marketing 231

17. Getting Out There: Stake Your Claim. 265

**How to Access Your Mind-Blowing Bonuses and
    Additional Resources 275**

Student and Client Testimonials 277

What Is a Healthcare Boss? 283

Acknowledgments. 289

About the Author 293

DEDICATION

To my wife, Nelly, your unwavering support and encouragement are almost superhuman. I could never do any of this without your compassion and trust. You are one of only a few things that make me truly happy. I am eternally grateful to have you in my life.

To my kiddos, Aria and Grayson, although you are cute little toddlers as I write this, you are the reason *why* I do what I do. If you read this down the road, remember: Protect your mind from toxic thoughts, live *your* life, stand up for what you believe in, always learn, take calculated risks, strive for greatness, and most importantly, be kind, be grateful, pray, and serve others. If you do these things, you will live a life of abundance. I love you both deeply. Watching you grow is one of the most rewarding things imaginable.

FOREWORD

When I quit my job in Commercial Real Estate back in 2012 to start a podcast, you can imagine I faced some fears … and some criticism. Even some of the best-known experts in the podcasting space shared doubts about my idea to start a daily podcast interviewing entrepreneurs. Not to mention my family—they also had some choice words about me leaving my partnership track behind to launch into an industry that a vast majority of the population didn't even know existed.

The fact is, the majority wants you to do what the majority does:

1. Earn a degree, (while burying yourself in debt);

2. Get a well-paying job, (so you can spend it all paying off your debt);

3. Be overworked and unhappy, (because most other people are, so why not?);

4. Rinse and repeat.

But if there's one thing I've learned over the past 10 years running one of the top business podcasts in the world, *Entrepreneurs On Fire*, it's this: You get to choose! You don't have to do what the majority does. And if you're willing to explore the opportunities available to you, then your dream life awaits. And that's exactly why you're here today, about to dive into an inspirational story and an informative playbook on how to launch your own clinic by Jason Duprat.

I first met Jason in person at my house in Puerto Rico. He took a chance, invested in himself, and flew down to spend the weekend with me, my partner Kate, and six other mastermind attendees.

I'll never forget Jason's time in the hot seat. He was the last hot seat of the day, and during it, he shared how miserable he was in his job—and also how passionate he was about his expertise. He talked about a world where he could help thousands of people, but on his own terms instead of someone else's. He shared his fears about not being able to support his family if he quit his job and what would happen if he went all in on his academy but failed.

After hearing Jason describe his situation and business momentum, I recommended—in no uncertain terms—that he quit his job and put all his focus into growing his Healthcare Entrepreneur Academy business. The mastermind ended for the day, and we dispersed.

The following day, Jason walked through my front door with a huge smile on his face. He looked me straight in the eyes and said, "I did it; I quit my job!" Jason's courage, strength, determination, and dedication to pursuing the life that he wanted to live are nothing short of inspiring. Because, guess what? It would have been way easier for Jason to fall back in line with the majority.

To believe that his only option was to stay at his job working for a giant healthcare corporation. To believe that if he was unhappy with his job and the long hours, the only solution was for him to go back to school, take on more debt, and get more degrees.

Do you believe that adding more letters after your name will lead you to jobs that provide the freedoms that you truly want? Do you believe that working for a giant healthcare corporation is your *only* path to success?

If you do, this book will prove otherwise.

Jason has spent the last five years inspiring thousands of healthcare professionals and helping them envision an alternative path to the burnout that corporate healthcare systems create—the path of entrepreneurship—which can be far more rewarding. Jason has created a movement of #HealthcareBosses, which has grown into a community of thousands of healthcare entrepreneurs helping and supporting others on their journey. This movement has exposed a world of opportunity that most healthcare professionals did not even know was possible.

Thanks to Jason's podcast and training programs, thousands are now operating their own clinics and other businesses. Imagine … No more overtime shifts or being forced to stay late, and no more missed holidays with the family. Imagine having weekends off, going on vacations, and attending your kids' games and events. All this can happen when you build a healthcare business that directly aligns with your personal and professional goals. Jason made a choice, and that was to follow his own path to success— without knowing the outcome.

Owning your own private clinic can transform your life, and no one knows this better than Jason.

This book will provide you with the knowledge you need to start the clinic of your dreams. Jason shares every mistake he made while starting his first clinic so that you can avoid the pitfalls and shortcut your path to success. The key is to take action, choose to forge your own destiny, and live life on your terms.

I'm sure you have a lot of questions about starting your own clinic. Lucky for you, Jason has the answers.

—John Lee Dumas,
Founder of *Entrepreneurs On Fire*

SECTION ONE

Making
the "Big" Decision

CHAPTER ONE

THE WAKE-UP CALL

"If you want something you've never had, you must be
willing to do something you've never done."

—*Thomas Jefferson*

y eyes flew open. My lungs reflexively attempted to expand rapidly. I tried to gasp for breath, but the pain wouldn't allow it. My back and chest were on fire.

I had jolted out of a sound sleep. Disoriented, I tried to roll over and sit up. The most excruciating pain I'd ever felt hit me like a Mack truck and flattened me back onto my pillow. I couldn't breathe.

"This could be a pulmonary embolism," my brain started telling me, but then it interrupted itself. "No, that doesn't make sense; I'd be tachycardic."

"Perhaps it's an aortic dissection," a second opinion said.

The first voice disagreed. "No, I think my blood pressure would be tanking by now." Apparently, my brain was having a consultation with itself.

"What about a myocardial infarction?"

"This seems like an atypical presentation. And why the hell does it hurt so much to breathe?"

Another voice showed up in my head, yelling over the other two. "Jason, get it together!" I had to snap out of it. "Get to the emergency room!" This guy was rational. I extended my arm out and reached for my wife. My hand found her torso, and I gave her a good shake.

"Babe, you need to take me to the hospital." My voice was scarcely above a whisper. My body was writhing in agony. "Something's wrong. My chest really hurts." I almost couldn't utter the words. Sweat was dripping down my face. Luckily, my wife is a light sleeper. In one fell swoop, she was out of bed, throwing on her shoes, and grabbing her purse and car keys.

The ride to the hospital felt like an eternity. Every time I tried to inhale, my body would stiffen, and my feet would kick out violently. It looked as if something was nipping at my heels, and I was trying to get away from it.

The pain was almost unbearable. My only saving grace was that the intensity of the pain would wax and wane. When it let up, I had just enough time to think for a half minute, get a little air, and prepare for the next round.

"Is this how it ends? Do I die at 35?" I asked myself in the moments when the pain abated slightly. "What about my wife? And the family we were supposed to create?"

"No." The rational guy was back. "That isn't happening," he said resolutely. "I'm not going to die. It's probably just a really bad muscle spasm."

—◦◦◦—

"Jason … Jason … " My wife's voice was like cool water on a fevered head. She was gently shaking my arm to wake me up. "Jason," she half-whispered, "Your test results are back. The doctor wants to talk to you." With Herculean effort, I slowly pulled my eyelids apart—first one and then the other. Dazed and confused, I looked around. I was in the emergency room.

"Okay. I'm awake." My words were soft and slightly slurred. I looked up and greeted the ER doctor. Trying to get my neurons to fire up was like trying to start an old car in the dead of winter in Alaska. Nevertheless, I was doing my best to muster the brain power to remember what had happened and decipher the mystery of why I was in a hospital bed. Only a few seconds went by as I got my bearings, but I could have sworn it was half an hour.

Morphine. That is what had happened. My wife told me the nurse had given me some morphine in my IV, and it had completely knocked me out. I had no idea how long it had been. She hadn't even given me the best stuff, but holy cow, it worked great. The relief didn't last long though. By the time they got me into an inpatient room, the pain was back up to a 10 out of 10. This experience was traumatic, made all the worse by being assigned a version of evil Nurse Ratched. But that's a different story …

At the time, I was working as a full-time nurse anesthetist at a hospital in Albuquerque. The money was great. Our plan had been for me to work at the hospital for three years and pay off all my student loans from anesthesia school. I had graduated with over six figures in college debt. I eventually paid all that off, but in doing so, I had to work an insane amount of hours.

My anesthesia department was short-staffed, like almost every anesthesia department in the country. They were constantly asking me to pick up extra shifts and stay late. Emergent cases would come in, so I couldn't leave.

Oftentimes, I'd get there at six in the morning to open up my operating room, and I wouldn't get home until after seven or eight at night. I also covered the high-risk labor and delivery unit. Those were 24-hour shifts. And I worked those three to four days a week. I practically lived at the hospital.

Let me paint a picture … The call room was a 10- by 12-foot cell. It had a tiny little bathroom and one window. Even if I wanted to break that window to get out, I couldn't. It didn't even open. It literally had wire mesh embedded in the glass. It was like a prison window.

The furniture looked like it was from the 1970s. The twin mattress reminded me of the one I used to sleep on in the spare room of my grandparents' house. You know the type. The ones with the coiled metal springs that had lost their ability to bounce back during the Carter Administration.

It was the kind of mattress where the center was so concave that you'd have to roll extra hard to unwedge yourself from the dip. And of course, those pointy springs would always poke me hardest when I was the most desperate for a few minutes of sleep, like those nights when I had been awake for over 20 hours straight, working in the busiest L&D unit in the city.

During those 24-hour shifts, I would get brief periods of "sleep" on that twin bed. I used quotation marks because it only laughably passed for sleep. You never knew when the next call was going to be, so even if there was a lull in the activity, I'd be on edge the whole time. Something or someone could walk through the door at any minute. I couldn't get too comfortable or too relaxed.

As a result of the stress of doing this for a year and a half, I ended up developing severe acid reflux and gastritis, which had gotten so bad that I developed peptic ulcers along with esophageal erosions. We had no idea why, but I had simultaneously developed rhabdomyolysis—and that's what landed me in the emergency room.

Needless to say, I was admitted. Later, when I was lying in that hospital bed alone at night, I began to feel depressed. I didn't see a light at the end of the tunnel. I knew that I'd have to return to work as soon as I was discharged.

I'd have to return to that exact same brutal schedule, and "sleep" in that exact same torture chamber of a call room. The hospital staff and managers would continue to guilt me into picking up shifts or staying late. And since I didn't want to be that guy who's not a team player or whose coworkers resented him because he wouldn't pitch in and cover shifts, I would continue to say yes.

My head started spinning like the hamster on the wheel that was my life. If I didn't find a way out, it would remain the same forever. I had already started to feel like a failure as a husband. I hardly ever saw my wife, and the time we did spend together, I was always completely exhausted and irritable.

I wasn't enjoying my life. I had lost my ambition to work out and stay fit and healthy. My mind was always in a fog from sleep deprivation. Even the rare times when I did get a day or two off in a row, it wasn't nearly enough time to fully recover.

What I always wanted was a career that I enjoyed, one that provided my family and me with a good living but still allowed me to spend time with them. Sure, I made a good income in the hospital, but what was the point if I couldn't enjoy it, be with the people I love, or do the things that added meaning to my life? I wanted a career that made me feel good about the work I was doing—something that allowed me to help people.

I laid my head back into my cheap, lumpy pillow with its starch-stiff pillowcase and closed my eyes. A past conversation popped into my head. A former ER physician had called me a year or so before, wanting to get my perspective on administering low-dose ketamine for mood disorders and chronic pain in an outpatient clinic. At that time, I had never heard of such a thing.

Since that phone call, the idea had been floating around in the back of my head. My mind started calculating. The average ER physician earned somewhere between $250,000 and $350,000 a year. That's not the kind of income you walk away from unless you can replace it.

I also knew that private clinics kept much better and more regular hours. If I were to follow suit and open my own clinic, maybe I could regain control of my time and actually get to see my family and friends in the evening, on weekends, and on holidays. Maybe that tunnel wasn't as endless as I thought. I saw a glimmer of light.

As soon as I was discharged, I started to do more research. After a few days, it was decided. I was going to become a healthcare entrepreneur and open up my own clinic. There was no way I was going to end up trapped, working the same endless hours at a hospital for the rest of my career.

The thought of continuing to sacrifice my nights, my weekends, my holidays, time with my wife, and ultimately my happiness, fueled me with motivation. I knew that sticking to the same path I was on would undoubtedly put me in the hospital again.

I even had a horror-inducing vision of becoming one of those fathers who was never there for his kids' games and important events. Or worse, and this made me feel sick in the pit of my stomach, I could become another divorce statistic.

I started researching what type of clinic I could own without having to go back to school for yet another degree or certification. It had to have low startup costs since I was still paying off my student loans. It also had to be something that didn't require a ton of my time since I would have to keep my hospital job for now. I needed a stable source of income as I got my business off the ground.

I researched a variety of different options. I knew that the type of clinic I chose would determine the hours and the lifestyle I would have. So I eliminated all the possibilities that didn't fit in with my ideal lifestyle or align with my interests. Ultimately, everything kept pointing back toward opening the same kind of clinic that the ER doctor had started: a ketamine therapy clinic.

As a nurse anesthetist, I administered ketamine on a regular basis, so it seemed like an obvious choice, but I also had another, more personal reason for wanting to pursue this path. Years earlier, my mom suffered from really severe depression. I helplessly watched her go through it. It got so bad that at one point, she couldn't even have a conversation without breaking out in tears.

All I knew to do was be supportive. I felt powerless. She was so depressed that she began to gain weight. This put her into a deep spiral, where the weight gain made her feel more depressed, so she would cope by eating. More weight gain caused worsening depression, and the spiral continued.

At the time, I had no idea how else to help her. But I now knew research was showing that ketamine could be used to treat mood disorders like treatment-resistant depression. The knowledge that I could potentially help patients in situations similar to my mom's became a driving force behind my desire to open a ketamine clinic.

These kinds of mental health issues are devastating. They destroy lives. And now I could offer people living with these hard-to-treat conditions the help they need. Everything about starting a ket-amine therapy clinic just felt right.

So my wife and I did the math. I had a choice—I could continue to provide anesthesia in a high-stress environment that destroyed my health and happiness, or I could provide ketamine therapy in a low-pressure environment where I could make my own sched-ule, take nights and weekends off, and go on vacation every once in a while. No brainer. But I was still a little hesitant. Was it too good to be true?

I didn't actually take the plunge until I saw a particular article published in the Journal of the American Medical Association (JAMA) Psychiatry. That was the deal-sealer for me. Before then, I had been thinking that maybe the idea was a little bit too risky because ketamine was not FDA-approved for treatment-resistant depression and the studies were still kind of sparse.

But then *JAMA Psychiatry* came out and said (I'm obviously para-phrasing here): "Hey, this is a treatment option that is working, we've reviewed the literature, and it needs more studies, but here is the protocol we would recommend for treating mood disorders."[1] *JAMA Psychiatry* is reputable and well-recognized, so when I saw this, I felt like it gave me the green light. Boom. It was time.

My first step was to start calling and texting everybody I knew, asking them if they knew anyone who had started a clinic. I kept

---

[1] Gerard Sanacora, MD, PhD; Mark A. Frye, MD; William McDonald, MD; et al. "A Consensus Statement on Ketamine in the Treatment of Mood Disorders," *JAMA Psychiatry,* (JAMA Network, April 1, 2017), https://jama-network.com/journals/jamapsychiatry/article-abstract/2605202.

coming up with dead ends. There were not very many advanced-practice nurses who had their own clinics back in 2017. I had a rough time finding any advice.

I tried looking for some sort of training program or certification course. I came up with absolutely nothing. Finally, I realized I would have to figure this out on my own. So that's what I did—figured it out as I went along. I started very small so as to be low-risk.

My first undergraduate degree was in business, so I felt fairly confident in my ability to handle that side of things. But I was making a lot of educated guesses on the business side, which meant I made plenty of mistakes.

I started calling all the different governmental departments in the area to learn more about the rules involved. I called the zoning department, the Board of Nursing, the Board of Pharmacy, and the Health Department, among others. I also searched all the relevant websites I could think of to ensure I was doing everything in a compliant manner.

I was able to fund a lot of the startup with cash flow from working. I started my clinic for $15,000, which is almost nothing. I already had my own malpractice insurance, which was one of the biggest expenses. The rest was relatively inexpensive. My wife and I did everything on a shoestring budget and with a lot of sweat equity.

It only took us about three months to open once we decided it was time. I kept my job for the first several months. But somehow the extra hours I was putting in for the clinic didn't feel like work, I was just so excited about it.

We started getting busier and busier and busier. Every step of the way, we were learning something new. If we ran into a wall, we would find a way over, under, around, or through it. We kept moving forward. Everything started to snowball. We built some great momentum.

Although we hit a few snags in the beginning, the pursuit turned out to be better than I ever imagined. I paid off all my startup expenses within the first three months, and shortly after that, I was able to match my hospital salary—working about half the hours.

We started to hire more staff, and I had more time off to pursue the things that I enjoyed. I was taking back control of my own schedule every day, little by little. I got to choose when or if I wanted to work. It took a good eight months, but I effectively made the transition from being an overworked, underappreciated nurse anesthetist to a successful clinic owner.

The clinic was so successful that clinicians started reaching out to me from all around the country, asking me how they could start their own clinics. Years later, I have been able to help hundreds of healthcare entrepreneurs either quit jobs they hate or reduce the hours they have to put into a system that overworked and underappreciated them. Jobs where they felt they weren't accomplishing anything truly meaningful. Now, they still care for patients, but they're in control and in a more impactful way.

I'm not here to give anyone the wrong impression. This is certainly not a get-rich-quick scheme. There is no easy button that you press and—*pow!*—you have a successful clinic. I can't guarantee that you're going to recoup your investment in three months like I did, nor can I guarantee that you'll make multiple six figures in your first year. You have to put in the work up front to get your clinic started and get your own momentum going, but the reward can be worth it a thousand times over.

There are many entrepreneurial opportunities out there for healthcare professionals to work in a way that makes them happy. If that's what you want, you'll have to change your paradigm to shift the way you think about things.

In school, we were taught that working in a corporate healthcare setting was the only thing that we could do. We were never even introduced to the possibility of starting our own business.

I am so grateful for that *one* conversation I had with the ER doctor all those years ago. I had no idea that he had planted a seed that would grow and drastically change the course and quality of my life. Now I'm on a mission to plant that seed in other people's minds.

You do not have to stay in a corporate healthcare setting to be a successful healthcare professional. There are other options out there. I'm going to tell you about the *one* that worked for me and many other healthcare professionals. It is possibly the easiest way to exit the corporate healthcare system. You get to use the same skill set you spent years honing but in a different setting where you have more autonomy and growth potential.

Some people are okay with working in the corporate healthcare setting. That's great, maybe starting a clinic isn't for them. But if you feel like you're living an existence that is less than it could be, showing up at work and going through the motions, or feeling overworked and overstressed, then starting a clinic might be for you.

The purpose of this book is to give you the foundation necessary for you to open a clinic and take control of your time and income. We will talk about the whole process: from when the idea is a figment of your imagination all the way to the birth of your clinic. There is a lot to cover.

We'll talk about what makes a self-pay clinic such a fantastic opportunity and why you would want to venture out and start one of your own. There are a lot of fears to overcome and myths to bust along the way. We'll go over the basics of planning your business, the rules and regulations you should be aware of, how to get everything up and running, and more. It sounds like a lot, I know. So let's get going.

CHAPTER TWO

THE MOST GRATIFYING BENEFITS OF SELF-PAY CLINICS

"The only limit to our realization of tomorrow will be our doubts of today."

—*Franklin D. Roosevelt*

Maya Angelou said, "If you are always trying to be normal, you will never know how amazing you can be." For most healthcare professionals, "normal" equates to working for a large healthcare organization. Often it means working for one that provides direct patient care and bills insurance for services.

Self-pay clinics (also called cash-based clinics or fee-for-service clinics) are different. They are clinics where patients pay out of pocket at the time of treatment. Mostly operating outside the control of insurance companies, this concept is a fantastic way to do business—not only because patient care is faster and unrestricted, but also because of the ease and flexibility it provides clinic owners and clinicians.

Clinic owners are plugging into this payment model to better meet customer needs without the delays, complexity, and costs associated with accepting payments from health insurance companies.

The focus of this book is on private clinics. A private clinic is owned by a licensed healthcare professional who is involved in the daily operations and often in patient care. In most states, private clinics can offer nearly any medical service. However, some require additional licenses or certification for invasive procedures such as surgery, interventional pain, or the administration of general anesthesia.

"But what's the big deal?" you might be asking yourself. "I have my education, I have my license, and I have a job. Why would I go through all the trouble of starting my own clinic if I already have that? It sounds like a massive pain." Sure does, but I have some pretty good answers for you.

First and foremost, owning your own clinic means you have more freedom, more autonomy, more command over your schedule, and you can uncap your income. At this point, I could stop and say "mic drop" and walk away, but if I did that, you'd be missing out on a myriad of other reasons to open your own practice.

Say Hello to Personal Fulfillment

What has been even more important to me than freedom and control is that I am helping people. For most of us healthcare professionals, everything we do is a result of our desire to help others. But with the expansion of corporate medicine over the years, and the ever-increasing production pressures, I found that I hardly ever felt like what I did was making any real difference.

When I was working at large hospitals and healthcare institutions, I felt like a cog in the wheel of an assembly-line healthcare system. Even though my anesthesia role is a vital part of the surgical process, I rarely left work feeling truly fulfilled. There was relentless pressure to provide care as quickly as possible. I never had the time to develop rapport and connection with my patients or their families.

Administrators were being pressured by executives to maximize the number of cases that could be done in a day, and they also had to meet metrics like on-time surgery starts, getting the next patient in the operating room in under 20 minutes, and a variety of other production-based goals. Speed and patient volume have become the primary foci of the healthcare system today.

Insurance reimbursements to hospitals and healthcare professionals have not been increasing anywhere near the rate of inflation. Take, for example, Medicare, Medicaid, and Tricare reimbursement rates. They are being frozen or cut. As a result, the only way for corporate medicine and healthcare workers to generate the same revenue year over year is to treat more patients. This pressure has put a tremendous amount of strain on healthcare workers who are already working extremely hard.

When I was working in the operating room every day, helping patients get through surgery, I could only help one patient at a time. Sometimes, when the surgeries were long, I could only care for one or two patients a day. This limited the number of people I was able to serve.

As a clinic owner, I was able to exponentially increase the number of patients I helped by building and leveraging a team. This means that by growing my clinic and hiring caring staff, I was responsible for serving many more patients each day.

I knew that I didn't have to be directly providing every patient's care, but through owning and managing the clinic, I was involved in changing each one of our patient's lives. My clinic served as a means for these people to be compassionately cared for and provided with treatments that could help them the most.

My impact and fulfillment were limited only by how much I wanted to grow my clinic; if I wanted to help more people, I could open a second or third clinic. The possibilities for expansion are limitless.

Say Bye-Bye to Insurance Companies

We all know what a pain it is to deal with insurance companies. They control the purse strings and therefore dictate what healthcare professionals can and can't do, oftentimes without regard to what is best for the patient. Having your own self-pay clinic gives you independence from insurance companies. You get to make your own calls in terms of the care you provide to your patients.

Here is a perfect example: a few months ago, I had to get another MRI for a low back injury that was caused by deadlifting in a CrossFit gym. My insurance said that I had to go and do six weeks of physical therapy before they would pay for it. Now, mind you, I had already done six weeks of physical therapy before the first MRI and it hadn't helped at all.

I had to deal with six more weeks of pain, wasted time, and co-pays, doing something I knew wouldn't work. Yet I was forced to complete another six weeks of physical therapy so the insurance would pay for the MRI that was ordered by a *specialized* physician and was necessary for him to make a diagnosis. Talk about a disservice to patients.

With a cash-based clinic, you have the freedom to provide the treatments that patients need. Providers in these practices don't have to put their patients through this hassle. If the provider orders a test or treatment, and the patient chooses to pay for it out-of-pocket, then the patient can get the care they need in a timely fashion. Providers can give the care that patients need without arbitrary hoops to jump through, time-wasting pre-authorizations, or refusals to pay.

Have you ever noticed that insurance companies seem to delay payments endlessly? The care is provided, the claim is submitted; it gets rejected for a multitude of reasons, and the claim has to be resubmitted. Wash-Rinse-Repeat. This is a never-ending cycle that wastes time and facility resources. Not to mention most billing companies will charge the clinic 5–7% of everything collected from the insurance companies.

With a self-pay clinic, you get paid right away. When you don't take insurance, you never have to deal with complicated billing codes or fight to get paid for the service you have already provided. Not having to deal with insurance is fantastic. It made me an even bigger believer in self-pay healthcare.

If you decide that you want to take insurance so that you can be affordable to all, I get it. But if this is the decision you make, you'd best save up several months' worth of business expenses before you open. Why? Well, when you're first getting enrolled as a provider in these insurance plans, it can take several months to get your first payment. This could result in serious cash-flow problems for a new clinic, and if you were not aware, cash-flow problems are the leading cause of small business failures. In fact, according to Score.org, 82% of small businesses fail because of cash flow issues.[2]

Don't Forget the Tax Benefits

Being a business owner also guarantees you certain leverage in terms of taxes. There is a two-tiered tax system in the US—one for business owners and one for W-2 employees. The majority of taxes in America are paid by W-2 employees. This is because a W-2 employee is required to pay taxes on 100% of their income. As a business owner, you only pay taxes on the business's net profit, not its income.

Let's dive a little deeper. You have your business's income, but you get to subtract all of the expenses that have anything to do with starting or operating the business. What is left is net profit. Because of this, you, as the clinic owner, will have the luxury of

---

[2] Brian Sutter, "The #1 Reason Small Businesses Fail—And How to Avoid It," SCORE Association, May 6, 2022, https://www.score.org/resource/blog-post/1-reason-small-businesses-fail-and-how-avoid-it.

not paying taxes on any expense required to generate business income.

Contrast that with a W-2 employee. A W-2 employee also has expenses related to earning their income, for example, the vehicle they use to drive to work, their cell phone, their uniforms, additional education, maintaining licenses and certifications, and the list of expenses goes on. The big difference is that as a W-2 employee, you don't get to deduct most of those expenses from your taxable income the way a business owner does.

Business owners have a lot of "owner benefits." For example, you can also take advantage of a company car for personal use, although the personal use portion is not tax-deductible, all expenses related to the business use are. There are a lot of tax-deductible business expenses that can also be used personally, like cell phones, internet, utilities, rent for office space, etc. The list goes on.

Owning your own business not only decreases your personal expenses but also decreases tax liabilities. The government provides these tax breaks because they want people like you and me to create and grow businesses that provide W-2 jobs to others. Those who are working well-paying W-2 jobs often pay a large percentage of their income in taxes, which is what funds the government.

It's Better for the Patient

Now, why would self-pay clinics be better for the patient? In a word, better quality service. Okay, that was three words, but any patient who frequents a cash-based clinic will tell you the service they receive is worth it. They get their appointments faster. They can get the treatments they need immediately without having to get insurance company approvals. It's easier to get telehealth visits, easier to get a prescription … everything about it is just easier and better for the patient.

Even though I have great health insurance, I personally go to a direct primary care clinic. I prefer it because I can usually get a same-day or next-day appointment, and I don't have to sit around wasting time in the waiting room. They also do teleconsults and give same-day prescriptions.

I pay a $69 monthly membership fee, which covers most of the basic services they offer and unlimited provider appointments. The providers are incredibly friendly, the patient evaluations are very thorough and never rushed, and I actually get treated like a human being. It's fantastic!

Contrast that with my previous insurance-based primary care provider, where I waited three weeks for an appointment and sat in the waiting room for over an hour. The staff and the patients were all irritable and unhappy. Not to mention my prescription took two days and repeated phone calls before it was finally called into the right pharmacy.

Why would anyone ever want to deal with that type of horrific service? I certainly don't. For me, $69 a month is a great value.

The passion that drives us healthcare practitioners is our desire to help people to the best of our ability; it's why we chose the field. A self-pay clinic helps us achieve that goal in an impactful way.

You get to help people not only by providing excellent medical and nursing services, but also by helping them bypass stressful and annoying steps in an insurance-based clinic. Everything in the process is simple and creates a seamless experience for the patient.

Today, there are even surgery centers around the country that only accept cash. They simply don't take insurance. They put a price for a knee replacement or any other surgery they offer right on their website. Going in, patients know exactly how much it will cost them.

With insurance providers footing the bill, patients can get burned even if they go into a hospital system that is in their insurance provider's network. The problem arises when the hospital has different subcontracted staffing groups. It's really common in anesthesia, emergency medicine, radiology, pathology, and even with inpatient labs.

Let me describe how this happens using anesthesia as an example. The unassuming patient has surgery at a particular facility because it is in-network. A month later, said patient gets a massive surprise bill associated with the cost of the surgery. "How can this be?" the bewildered and still-recovering patient asks. "The hospital is in my network!"

After several aggravating back-and-forths with the hospital's billing department and their insurance company, the patient figures it out. The hospital hired an outside anesthesia group and that group is privately owned and operated. Those anesthesia providers were not in-network with the patient's insurance.

The same thing often happens in the emergency room. A patient can look up that particular location, and it says they're in-network, but they have ER providers, radiology departments, or even lab services that are subcontracted out. So a patient can be treated by an in-network hospital and still end up with huge ER provider, lab, or even radiology bills at the end of whatever distressing incident brought them there in the first place.

It's ludicrous and has gone on for decades. US healthcare is the only industry where it is not common practice to tell a patient what they will pay for a service prior to having the service provided. Thank God, politicians are finally starting to act on this wildly unethical billing practice. A practice that our corporate healthcare systems actively lobby to keep in place. Disgraceful. When a patient comes to a cash-based clinic, sure, they're paying out of pocket—but they know exactly what they're purchasing and exactly what they're spending.

Another College Degree Is Not the Answer

As medical and health professionals, we are indoctrinated with the idea that to advance in our field or be worthy of a pay raise, we have to continue to get more degrees and credentials. The truth is, while we do need extensive schooling for what we do, additional schooling is not always better.

If your goal is to continue to specialize in more precise areas of healthcare or research and to continue being an employee rather than a business owner, then by all means go back to school and keep getting more degrees. But if you're reading this book, my guess is that's not what you want.

To my way of thinking, more degrees typically equal more debt, more time not making the money you want to make, and less freedom. If your goal is to earn a good living while still being able to enjoy life and do the things that you want to do while serving patients and making a positive impact, then going back to school is a long, expensive, and inefficient way to get there. Trust me, I tried that route.

After I opened my clinic, I didn't feel 100% confident in my ability to run a business, so I thought getting an MBA would help me out. After enrolling in an MBA program, I quickly realized that an MBA focused almost exclusively on teaching students how to be good managers in *large* companies. The university system was still teaching me how to work for someone else and make that someone else profit.

And yet, I persisted and ultimately finished the MBA program. I kept hoping that I would eventually learn something that would help me as an entrepreneur and clinic owner, but I never did, and that came at a cost: the opportunity cost.

As a business owner, you always have to look at both the benefits and costs of your actions, inactions, and choices. When you factor in the opportunity cost of getting a degree and tack that on to the cost of tuition, it often makes many degrees a terrible investment.

In my case, choosing to get my MBA cost me time and money that I could have used to grow my practice even faster. It took me over two and a half years to earn my MBA. I spent about 15 hours a week listening to lectures, reading, and completing assignments for my classes. If I had taken the $26,000 I spent on my Master's degree, along with those 1,950 hours spent, and invested all of that time and money back into my business, it would have catapulted us light years ahead.

Once you become an entrepreneur, you will learn the importance of making decisions based on the return on investment (ROI) and not on what others have brainwashed you into believing. Imagine starting another degree at a university and, within three months, being able to make money from what you've learned. And I don't mean getting a job on campus where you make $10 an hour working as a teaching assistant. I'm talking about real money—money that would rival or exceed your current salary. It sounds too good to be true, doesn't it?

After earning four degrees from various universities—two bachelor's and two master's degrees—I have yet to encounter any degree that comes close to being able to earn you a good salary within a few months of starting. What *did* start making me good money within three months of starting, however, was launching my own clinic.

I can tell you firsthand, without any hesitation, that you do not need an MBA or any fancy business degree to be a successful entrepreneur. With substantial sweat equity, I was able to open my clinic for less than $15,000. Most advanced degrees are 2–5 times more expensive. And I can promise you that none of them can earn you a great income faster than opening your own clinic.

Who Can Own a Self-Pay Clinic?

This is probably the most common question I get asked. The answer is both simple and super-technical. The simple answer is: "Anyone." That's right, anyone. It's simply a matter of how you structure it—the structuring is the super-technical part. The way you structure your clinic ultimately depends on the state you're in and the type of professional license you have.

The details in this section can get complex. It requires a thorough understanding of state laws and scopes of practice. The intricacies are outside the purview of this book, but I will do my best to provide a clear overview.

For the purposes of this book, the definition of a "provider," as in "healthcare provider," is a licensed healthcare professional that can evaluate patients, prescribe treatment plans, prescribe and administer medications, and refer patients to other healthcare specialists. There are several types of providers in the United States.

Physicians, such as Medical Doctors (MDs) and Doctors of Osteopathy (DOs) are the providers most people are familiar with. In addition, there are Physician Associates (PAs), formerly called Physician Assistants, and there are Advanced Practice Registered Nurses (APRNs).

As of the writing of this book, Physician Associates are required to be supervised by a physician in all US states and territories. Depending on the state, APRNs may be able to practice independently of a physician or they may be required to collaborate with a physician (the majority of states are now like this). In the most restrictive states, APRNs are required to be supervised by a physician.

For APRNs, each state has a different way of regulating the clinic operations and ownership details. Not all states even use the term or credential "APRN" yet, so let's get clear on who this encompasses.

An APRN is a registered nurse who has also completed a master's or doctoral degree, completed a minimum number of hours of nurse residency and clinical hands-on-training, and passed a licensing board examination to become one of the following types of advanced-practice nurses: a family nurse practitioner, certified registered nurse anesthetist, clinical nurse specialist, acute care nurse practitioner, psychiatric mental health nurse practitioner, gerontological nurse practitioner, or nurse midwife.

An APRN can evaluate patients, prescribe treatment plans, prescribe and administer medications, and provide most, if not all, of the services that a physician provides.

What varies state-by-state for APRNs is the level of physician oversight required for them to provide care. An APRN who is licensed in an independent practice state can start, own, and operate a private practice or medical clinic without any physician involvement. In a non-independent practice state, the APRN would need to hire or partner with a physician, or possibly another APRN, whose specialization allows them to practice independently.

If you are *not* a provider, there are more steps to getting a clinic started, but it is still very possible. We have helped several dozen of our non-provider students start their own clinics. The key takeaway for non-providers, such as registered nurses or other healthcare professionals, is that they will need to hire or partner with a provider. In some states with corporate practice of medicine restrictions, this may mean sharing ownership equity with the provider.

It is critically important to understand that a provider *must* evaluate patients, prescribe treatment plans, and prescribe any medications. Once that has been completed, the other staff in the clinic, such as the registered nurses, can provide care and administer medications or treatments ordered by the provider.

Once you understand these key concepts and learn what the various license types are authorized to do according to their scopes of practice, building a clinic that meets your goals is straightforward. Don't rush over this part of your planning, you must ensure that everyone working in the practice is only providing the care authorized in their scope of practice.

Almost anyone can own a healthcare business, and in many states, you don't even need a healthcare degree to own a clinic, hospital, or healthcare facility. There are a few states that have some exceptions, like California, but there are almost always legal workarounds.

For example, an entrepreneur might want to start a clinic, but they wouldn't be able to start a private practice because they're not licensed healthcare professionals. They could still start the exact same clinic, offering the exact same services, but the terminology and the rules may be different.

Oftentimes, they will have to jump through additional business licensing and regulatory hoops because they don't know about standards of care, don't understand how to dispose of medical waste, how to order pharmaceuticals, how a nurse or a doctor functions, and all sorts of other healthcare-related technicalities. However, I am writing this book to help licensed healthcare professionals, so I won't be going into all the details for non-licensed individuals here.

There are states (Texas, for example) that only allow physicians to use the term "medical" clinic, but even then, there are workarounds. If you are an APRN, you can call your practice a "wellness clinic" or "health clinic" or "primary care clinic." This is one of the times (there are many) when I will tell you to consult with an experienced attorney in your state. Part of their role in your startup is to advise you of the state requirements and how you can meet them.

In many cases, all the licensed clinic owner needs to do is ensure the proper independent provider works for the business or is a part owner. At my clinic in New Mexico, that meant I had to hire an independent family nurse practitioner to evaluate patients, prescribe treatment plans, and prescribe medications by writing orders.

In other states, a physician might have to "supervise" the provider who writes those orders. APRNs who are licensed and live in a fully independent practice state will be able to independently write their own orders.

I do want to make it clear—anybody performing any procedures in a clinic has to be a licensed healthcare professional, and their license has to allow them to do whatever tasks they're doing.

You Can Start Small

A few years before I started my clinic, I was really into CrossFit®. CrossFit has a brilliant business model. They only have a few pieces of cardio equipment and no weight machines, which are the biggest startup costs for a typical gym.

Instead, CrossFit gyms have high-intensity exercise training programs for small groups. They mostly use dumbbells, barbells, and bodyweight exercises, so the equipment costs are minimal, and depending on the size of the gym, they may only need enough equipment for fifteen to twenty people at a time. This also means they don't need a lot of space.

In addition, because classes are run in groups, people don't come in and out whenever they want; the owner has total control over when they're open and when the classes are scheduled. When groups aren't in session, you don't need any staff around. So that keeps labor costs low too.

Initially, I thought opening a private clinic and purchasing everything I needed would be really expensive because, as a nurse anesthetist, I spent most of my time in an operating room. And, as you know, surgery is very costly. There's the surgeon's salary and the salaries for the rest of the staff, which includes RNs, surgical assistants, anesthesia personnel, anesthesia machine, surgical lights, the operating table, and all the other equipment and supplies. So I mistakenly let this false belief hold me back as I pondered all different kinds of clinics.

But then the business model of that CrossFit gym came to mind. What if I could come up with a practice idea that didn't require tons of expensive equipment? That meant anything like urgent care, dialysis, or a clinic that offered expensive treatments—like cosmetic surgery or laser treatments—was out of the question. All of these required a lot of expensive equipment, long hours of operation, and a lot of staff.

When I started thinking about services I could offer, I listed options that were effective, in-demand, and didn't require a large amount of capital to get into. It dawned on me that the IV ketamine and IV nutritional therapy clinic model was similar to the CrossFit gym model.

Unlike having a clinic that might require surgical suites and expensive laser equipment, I realized that with IV infusions, specifically ketamine infusions, I could start with one specific treatment that needed minimal equipment. It only required a monitor, an infusion pump, and a chair. That cut down on start-up costs dramatically.

Patients had to make an appointment, so I didn't need to have the clinic open all day. I was highly trained and experienced with ketamine and was great at IV insertions. Plus, I felt personally connected to my ideal patients because of my mom's history of depression. All of this added up to a business model that was imminently doable for me. It was a simple model and a low-investment type of clinic.

A clinic is a business; it enables you to render products and/or services to customers and makes a profit in the process. A clinic's business model consists of the products and services you offer, how you plan to deliver them, and how you are going to generate revenue from those particular products or services. To run a successful business for the long term, you need to understand the services that best align with your future goals.

There are about as many different clinic services as there are clinic owners. Throughout this book, we are going to use three popular self-pay clinic services as examples: IV therapy, Ketamine therapy, and Med Spas. Some of the other common self-pay services include direct primary care, urgent care, weight loss, hormone replacement, functional medicine, and surgical centers.

IV Therapy

IV therapy is a service that involves a healthcare professional inserting an intravenous (IV) catheter into a patient's vein and administering an infusion of fluid or a fluid combined with a pharmacological substance. These substances are usually medications, vitamins, minerals, chelating agents, or antioxidants.

You'll hear it called a bunch of different names. There's IV therapy, IV hydration, IV nutritional therapy, and IV hydration therapy, but they're all synonymous. Our training programs have dozens of hours of course content on the various clinical uses of IV therapy, along with protocols and in-depth clinic start-up content. There is far too much to discuss in this book, but let's cover a few examples of different types of IV therapies.

IV therapy can be offered as a simple treatment for hangover symptoms. I have taught several business workshops in Las Vegas, and IV therapy services are very popular in this city. This tends to result from those who overindulge in adult beverages and are seeking a faster recovery with some IV fluids, medications such as Zofran and Toradol, as well as a rapid influx of vitamins and minerals.

Some IV clinicians specialize in treatments like chelation and administer pharmaceuticals that bind to toxins in your body to aid in their elimination. Other IV service providers specialize in ozone therapy. Ozone is an alternative treatment with some limited research behind it that shows it may be able to boost the immune system.

There are avid customers of IV therapy clinics. One group is the health and wellness optimization crowd—especially the athletes. They may run marathons, compete in triathlons, be CrossFit competitors, or be any other type of dedicated athlete, but they often seek rapid rehydration due to large depletions of fluid and electrolytes from intense training or competitions. B-vitamin injections are also popular among athletes and even non-athletes since the B vitamins support metabolism and energy.

Yet another group of people who might come in for IV therapy are those who have medical conditions that impair their ability to absorb oral supplements or oral nutrition. They might be patients with gastrointestinal (GI) disorders or post-surgical GI patients. Others may seek treatment because they would like vitamins dosed at a level that isn't well tolerated through oral consumption, such as high-dose vitamin C.

Ketamine Therapy

Ketamine is a medication that has traditionally been used as an anesthetic and analgesic for medical procedures and surgery.

More recently, it has been used off-label as a treatment for depression and other mental health conditions.

Ketamine infusion therapy involves administering low doses of the drug intravenously over the course of several weeks or months. The exact protocol for ketamine therapy may vary depending on the specific condition being treated and the healthcare provider administering the treatment. Although IV ketamine is the most researched route of administration, some clinics are also administering ketamine IM, sublingual, or intranasal.

Studies demonstrate that ketamine has rapid antidepressant effects. It can also be helpful for rapidly alleviating suicidal ideations and decreasing symptoms of other psychiatric conditions. However, more research is needed to understand the risks of its long-term use and to determine the optimal protocol and route of administration.

Nevertheless, this treatment has undoubtedly provided relief for tens of thousands of patients in recent years. It is important to note that ketamine can cause side effects, including hallucinations, dissociation, increased blood pressure and heart rate, and should be administered by personnel trained in its use.

Med Spa

Med Spa is short for medical spa and is a type of healthcare facility that combines traditional medical treatments with spa services. Medical spas are often overseen by a healthcare provider and offer a range of treatments that are designed to improve the health and appearance of the skin.

Medical spas may offer a variety of services, including facials, chemical peels, microdermabrasion, laser hair removal, injectable treatments such as Botox® and fillers, or even invasive surgical procedures. These treatments may be performed by licensed medical professionals such as physicians, APRNs, PAs, nurses, or aestheticians.

Mixed Service Models

There are specialty clinics that choose to provide a single service as well as offer a variety of complementary services. There is no one-size-fits-all recipe for success, but I personally recommend starting with a limited number of services. It can get very overwhelming to try to open a clinic that offers a multitude of different services. Not to mention, marketing a large number of services is extremely difficult and costly.

Returning to ketamine as a case study, running a ketamine clinic as a specialty practice can be a profitable service model. Most of the initial ketamine clinics in the US only offered ketamine therapy, but as the literature supporting ketamine therapy grows, so does clinician awareness. And as the field of ketamine therapy continues to mature, we're starting to see a variety of different clinics also add ketamine therapy into their already existing practices.

Med Spas are an example of those starting to offer ketamine therapy. It's easier for them because they already have a spa-like atmosphere, and many are providing IV infusions as an ancillary service. It's a pretty straightforward add-on for them. They simply need to have the appropriate staff members complete a

CE- or CME-approved training, purchase a cardiac monitor, and then add ketamine therapy into their practice model.

Other add-on services for a Med Spa might be eyelash extensions, micro-needling, microblading, teeth whitening, laser tattoo removal, or non-invasive body contouring.

When I first opened my clinic, my idea was to create a specialized practice where I started with ketamine infusion therapy. Since then, a whole world has opened up to me, and I don't just mean all the possible services that can be offered in one's clinic.

As a result of starting, growing, and ultimately selling my first successful clinic, an opportunity that I never even expected came my way. I began helping healthcare professionals all over the country who were looking for guidance in starting their own clinics. It ultimately resulted in me creating several training programs under an overarching brand called the Healthcare Entrepreneur Academy. These training programs include the Ketamine Academy, the IV Therapy Academy, and the Med Spa Launch Academy. Depending on when you read this book, we may have even more training programs.

Now I even have the privilege of hosting a podcast, aptly named the *Healthcare Entrepreneur Academy* podcast. This show is dedicated to educating, motivating, and inspiring other healthcare professionals along their entrepreneurial journey. To learn more, you can head over to:

jasonduprat.com/book

Helping other healthcare professionals start and grow their own clinics and other businesses has been one of the most rewarding things that I have experienced. I love the business I have created, and it goes to show that if you follow your interests and strive to get great at what you do, opportunity is right around the corner.

CHAPTER THREE

MINDSET: THE "HOLY GRAIL"

*"Whether you think you can,
or you think you can't—you're right."*

—*Henry Ford*

Let's be honest, fear can dominate your life, and sometimes you don't even know it. It can come in many forms and inhibit your progress. It can be in those rationalizations, the "I'll do it laters," and the lack of faith in your own abilities that keeps you from even getting started.

I implore you: do not let fear hold you back from the life of your dreams. Instead, study it, understand it, and learn to control it so you'll be able to achieve greater things in your life.

I am neither a life coach nor a motivational speaker, but I know for a fact that a negative mindset—pessimistic thought patterns, fear, and self-doubt—can and will hold you back from your peak level of success, whatever that looks like for you.

But how do you counter a mindset that has been instilled in your brain by society since you were little? I recommend you find podcasts, books, coaches, conferences, courses, and masterminds to help retrain your way of thinking. Always surround yourself with top performers. Align yourself with those who can push you forward and pull you upward.

Motivational speaker Jim Rohn famously said, "You are the average of the five people you spend the most time with." If you hang around with people who only talk about the latest episode of their favorite Netflix series, that will be all *you* talk about.

If you cultivate friendships with people who have achieved great things—that you also hope to attain in the future—you will always be challenged to grow and will have connections who can help you accomplish your goals.

Overcome Your Fears and Limiting Beliefs

The doors were unlocked. The staff was there. The equipment was in place. We had gone through months of blood, sweat, and tears to open the clinic, and there we stood, behind the front desk, looking at an empty waiting room. The appointment calendar was completely blank. I could hear my heartbeat in my ears. Desperate hopes for a walk-in patient danced around in my brain.

Thankfully, that event never happened. It was merely an image created in my mind by fear. But it was so pervasive and powerful that it was able to plant worst-case scenario after worst-case scenario in my mind.

Those images tried to play out in my head often enough that I started to doubt if starting a clinic would be the right move. It even made me take another look at keeping my hospital job. It was at least secure, right? The paycheck would always be there. But so would the stress, the long hours, and the terrible work schedule, not to mention my mental and physical exhaustion.

It was a discomfort contest. Which was worse? The everlasting burnout I was experiencing at my job? Or the idea that I could fail, take a blow to my ego, and go back to work in a hospital? We are all inclined to move away from those things that we perceive to cause us the *most* discomfort.

Luckily for me, I was still working full-time when I was opening my clinic, which reminded me every day how unhappy I was. I felt like I was in the movie *Groundhog Day*: wake up before sunrise, punch the time clock, and work until dark. Head home, eat, shower, sleep, repeat. Over and over and over. I had to get out of that cycle.

I *had* to keep going with my plans for starting the practice while I still had some energy and motivation left in me. I couldn't let myself succumb to the hamster wheel of an ordinary life without a fight.

When I first opened my clinic, I quickly discovered that my fears were completely unfounded. I already had patients who had booked appointments weeks prior. Many of these people were suffering from treatment-resistant depression, chronic pain, and other conditions. They had been researching ketamine for months or even years. And they were waiting with anticipation for someone like me to open up a clinic close enough to them.

I had some initial administrative and regulatory challenges, but my clinic growth was nearly doubling month after month for the first six or seven months. We had some patients fly in from across the country because we were the most affordable clinic in the country when we started. Many of my patients drove four to six hours to get treatment at my clinic.

We started lean and grew so quickly that, as I said, I made back my entire startup investment in about three months of being open. We used the cash flow from the business to double the number of infusion chairs. We built a private infusion room and made other investments to improve the patient experience.

After a few months, I was consistently generating thousands of dollars in net profit every month. This quickly rose to $10K in monthly profit and continued growing until it matched, then surpassed, the monthly income I was earning as a 1099 anesthesia provider.

Within nine months, I had exceeded my previous year's income, added a tremendous asset to my portfolio, and helped hundreds of patients find symptom relief when everything else they had tried failed. All of that happened because I didn't give in to my fear. I chose to push those negative voices out of my mind, while taking small actions every day to move toward my clinic ownership goals.

Being scared about a huge life change like this is normal. It means you're a thoughtful and meticulous decision-maker. The key is to recognize the fear and use it to help you take action. For example, the fear of having an empty clinic because you don't know how to attract new patients makes you want to invest time in learning about clinic marketing and patient retention.

You can and should mitigate risks where they can be mitigated. This is best done through education and investing in expert guidance. Fear is often a fear of the unknown. By educating yourself, you will quell some of those uncertainties. And by seeking expert guidance, you can rest assured that there is almost always someone there who has successfully done it before, ready to answer questions and have your back anytime you need it.

Hands down, the most common reason people don't succeed is that they let fear control their thoughts. Fear is one of the biggest hurdles to overcome. For any chance of success, it is vital that you have a resilient mindset, overcome fear, and have faith that you can start and grow a successful clinic.

I don't recall exactly where I first heard these few lines, but they have stuck with me for years because they are so impactful. *Your circumstances influence your thoughts. Your thoughts create your feelings. Your feelings determine your actions. Your actions forge your future.* Your future starts in your mind. Fear is part of the normal response to a change in your circumstances.

If you haven't started a clinic from scratch, operated a business, or managed a team of employees, all of this may seem intimidating at first. With so many new things to learn and implement, the most important thing is to recognize that fearful thoughts are totally normal. You can't control the thoughts that pop into your mind, but you *can* control how long you let them stay there.

Fear is a deeply embedded instinct within our DNA and serves the awesome purpose of keeping us alive. Fear provokes the fight-or-flight response to protect us from dangerous or unfamiliar situations. This biological fight-or-flight reaction is a God-given response, meant to save us from physically harmful involvements so we can survive and procreate. This response is crucial in life-or-death situations, like in times of war or back when humans lived in the wilderness.

In today's modern world, we aren't running from tigers, but we still have that reaction to perceived threats. Now, rather than saving our lives, fear that is unrecognized and uncontrolled has become a significant barrier to success for many people. All you have to do is recognize it, mitigate any real risks, and keep pushing forward.

The Zone of Mediocrity

When you feel yourself coasting or losing your passion, it's most likely because you're not challenging yourself. You are stuck in a rut. That rut is called your comfort zone. It is human nature to want to stay within the boundaries of your comfort zone. Everything in this zone is, by its very nature, comfortable; it is safe and cozy. The average human mind operating here is free from risk or challenge.

While that may sound nice, it is also true that comfort leads to complacency. Complacency leads to stagnation. Stagnation leads to unhappiness. Humans are not designed to be stagnant. We are designed to grow and thrive.

You will never find the next level of happiness, success, and freedom within your comfort zone. To reach the next level, you must be willing to move out of its confinement—to venture forth, leaving complacency behind.

There are two simple truths about comfort zones you should be aware of. These two things are why your future happiness and success will never be found there:

1. "Comfort zone" is synonymous with "zone of mediocrity."
2. Nothing truly great was ever achieved by anyone who stayed within their comfort zone.

If you study history books to learn from thousands of examples of world-class achievers and high-level performers, be it in business, sports, or innovation, you will see that great successes were always accomplished when people pushed themselves past the things they found easy to do.

Moving past these things takes a conscious effort. You have to push yourself upward, step by step, to reach the next level. If you don't, life will simply pass you by. Failure to leave your comfort zone often results in the withering away of your dreams. Ultimately, it lessens the motivation to live an abundant and fulfilled life. Instead, its inhabitants dwell in mediocrity.

Rather than wake up and confront the numbness, they often find relief by distracting themselves with endless hours of video games or binging on Netflix. They bury themselves in unproductive work or spend thousands of hours watching, studying, and memorizing stats about their favorite sports or athletes. They will do nearly anything to avoid the reality they created for themselves.

Let me ask you a question. How happy are you with your life and career right now? Seriously, take a minute and think about it.

Now, ask yourself:

- Do I wake up every day looking forward to going to work?
- Am I unable to sleep at night because I am excited about something I get to do or work on at my day job?
- Do I consider work to be work?
- Is work fun?
- Is work something I would do for little or no money if I could?

If this is you, congratulations! You, my friend, are likely living a life of purpose, growth, and fulfillment. But if you didn't answer "yes" to many of those questions, then ask yourself:

- Do I wake up dreading the next shift?
- Do I start counting down the hours almost immediately after I arrive at my job?
- Do I catch my mind wandering and fantasize about other opportunities or careers?
- Do I come home after every shift completely exhausted, leaving only the worst parts of myself—the leftovers—for my family?
- Do I get angry or frustrated when I am requested to work later than I was originally scheduled?
- Do I miss a substantial number of holidays or family events because of my work schedule?

- Do my kids or my spouse feel as though things aren't as they should be?
- Do I think my relationships are suffering because I'm always at work?

If this is you, wake up and get out! If you don't, 20 years from now, you will realize that the best part of your life has flown by and you have gotten nowhere—that you had given up on your dreams decades ago.

Change can begin now. Start studying how to shift any negative thought patterns. Your mind is the key determinant of your success. Your thoughts are born from your subconscious reactions, habits, and thought processes. Learn how to recognize the wrong ones and replace them with positive thoughts that will move you forward.

Myth-Busting: The Most Common

Laird Hamilton said it best: "Make sure your worst enemy is not living between your own two ears." You may find that one of the first things your psyche does to keep you from venturing out of your comfort zone is to start formulating myths, excuses, or even lies about why you can't do it. That's okay. Your psyche is just trying to protect you.

But, much like a helicopter parent is well-meaning, this kind of "protection" will only foster dependency and inaction. If you're reading this book, you are likely an action-taker. Don't lose that valuable trait.

So what are the things keeping you from jumping headfirst into starting your own clinic? After educating and coaching hundreds of healthcare professionals, I have a pretty good idea.

I know the most common myths clients tend to tell themselves. And I have found that there are nine. You're already thinking of one, some, or all of them, so let's just address them head-on.

Myth #1: I Need to Have Some Kind of Business Experience Before I Can Own My Own Clinic

Having pre-existing business experience before opening your own clinic would be useful, but it is not a necessity. Do you think Steve Jobs or Jeff Bezos had prior business management experience when they started Apple or Amazon in their garage? Steve Jobs dropped out of college and took a trip to India before eventually starting Apple. All he had as far as business experience was a summer internship at Hewlett-Packard while he was in high school. Jeff Bezos was a computer engineer by trade before starting Amazon.

The reason that somebody becomes a successful business owner isn't that they have experience starting a business. They create a successful business because they see a problem in the world and choose to offer a great solution. Then they learn the things they need to know about business—in the trenches—as they need to learn them. They are also great at finding people with experience to guide them or join their team.

Myth #2: Starting a Private Clinic Is Really Expensive

I'm often a bit baffled whenever I hear people say that starting a private clinic is really expensive. The people who say this are usually looking to get another degree, which can cost another $30,000 to $50,000, or more. As healthcare professionals, many of us spent years in college. Many have spent over a decade learning their craft.

We talked about this earlier, but it bears repeating … We have been indoctrinated into the concept that more college and more degrees equals more money and more status. But the reality is that when I started my clinic in 2017, it cost me less than $15,000 to open. That's less than a single semester at many universities.

Not everyone lives in an area or chooses a business model where it's feasible to open a clinic for under $15,000. A reasonable start-up number these days is $20,000–$25,000. Within the first year of opening my clinic, my business was *netting* over $150,000. That's after reinvesting extensively for future growth.

Considering that the small business association says that the average business loses money for the first two to three years, a profit of well over six figures in the first year is almost supernatural in entrepreneur-land. Starting a clinic allowed me to earn my first $150,000 two years faster than getting another degree would have.

And my story isn't special or rare. I know of several clinic owners who net well over $250,000 a year in their first couple of years. So if I started a clinic tomorrow and it somehow costs me $100,000, I could *still* easily recoup all my startup expenses and generate a profit in far less time than it took me to earn a master's degree that may or may not even allow me to earn six figures or multiple six figures.

The benefit doesn't stop there. By working as a nurse anesthetist, I was trading my time for dollars. If I didn't work, I didn't get paid. At some point, the number of hours I could work reached a peak. At the point I could no longer work any more hours, my income was capped.

However, with a clinic, you can begin to use leverage. In business, leverage allows you to earn money without trading your time for it. By hiring and building a team, you are leveraging the ability of your clinic staff to work and provide patient care when you can't (or don't want to), therefore your income is no longer capped at the maximum amount of hours you can physically work.

What's more, your income in this business is almost infinitely scalable. There are business owners who own a dozen or more clinics. Some have grown by selling a franchise. You're limited only by how you limit yourself.

Myth #3: Business Owners Work All the Time and Have Even Worse Hours Than Healthcare Professionals

Okay … this myth *can* be true. It's often true that when putting in the initial work to get the business off the ground, many business owners work extensively and have even worse hours than healthcare professionals. Of course, it's true for many ongoing business owners as well. But here's a little secret: it's their own fault if they let that go on for too long.

Think of a business owner as a conductor of an orchestra. It's not the conductor's job to play the violin, the cello, the clarinet, and every other instrument. It's their job to ensure that all the instruments play in sync. Being a business owner is the same.

Your long-term job isn't to be the accountant, the marketer, the receptionist, the janitor, and the one who treats patients. Now, you may have to do all those things initially, but if you try to do all of that for an extended period, you'll get burned out quickly. You aren't really running a business at that point. You just own a job.

Do you think Jeff Bezos is in the warehouse picking orders and then putting them in a box? Do you think Steve Jobs was in the factories assembling iPhones when he was the CEO of Apple? Absolutely not.

Business owners are busy making sure that all of the parts work together in unison so the entire business runs smoothly. They find people who are better than themselves at all of those different tasks, hire them, give them direction, and then let them do what they do best.

I hate dealing with day-to-day finances for my business, so I hired an accountant to take that off my hands. Not only did that make me immensely happier, but it also freed me up to work on growing my clinic.

As soon as I could, I hired a receptionist to greet people as they enter, set appointments, call patients, and follow up with them after their treatment. This freed up even more of my time and left me able to continue growing my practice.

As we grew, I hired other nurses and nurse practitioners to provide treatments to patients. When they came in, this freed up even *more* of my time.

At that point, less than a year into the business, things were going so well that I had no problem taking time off to spend with my family, go to the gym, and return to doing some of the things that made me happy again. Before I knew it, I was no longer working weekends and took all major holidays off because I closed the clinic on holidays.

Myth #4: I Need to Quit My Current Job to Start a New Business

When I was first looking into starting a clinic, I was concerned because I thought I'd have to quit my job and wouldn't be able to pay my student loans, my mortgage, or my other bills. Quitting my job was out of the question.

That was one of the things I found so attractive about starting my clinic. I ran it by appointment only and I only accepted appointments when I was not working at the hospital. This had multiple benefits. The first one was that I could keep my current job and income.

It also meant I could reinvest a large percentage of the money I was making from my clinic into paying off my startup costs, purchasing the equipment I needed to expand the practice, and tucking away the rest as emergency savings.

That way, when I was ready to quit my job, I had a very nice cushion and could easily pay myself an excellent salary. It also allowed me to grow my business at a pace that I was comfortable with. I never felt like I had to rush the process just to pay the bills.

I built a client base, a referral network, and a marketing system over several months. So I knew that when I did make the leap, I would be able to consistently and reliably bring in new patients and make a steady income.

Myth #5: I Don't Have the Time to Run a Business

I completely understand why you might think that you don't have enough time to start a business. Between work and family obligations, you may feel like you're already spread thin. I get it, trust me. I was averaging 60 to 70 hours a week at the hospital when I first started my clinic. Those crazy hours were exactly why I *had* to open my clinic. I could not keep that crazy schedule. It was a one-way train to a miserable life.

Not having a lot of time was actually a huge benefit for me. I know it sounds counter-intuitive, but have you ever heard of "Parkinson's Law?" It is the adage that states: "Work expands to fill the time available." Put another way, it will take you however long you have, to do whatever it is that you need to do. The truth is that we could accomplish in 30 minutes what would normally take two hours to do if we just put a little pressure on ourselves to get it done.

How often are you distracted for five minutes here, ten minutes there by social media, another app on your phone, or some Netflix series? How many hours do you think that adds up to? I can assure you that it's probably a lot more than you would guess.

What I did was use the downtime I had at work. If I had half an hour or an hour between surgeries, I would read another research article, call about a clinic space that I was interested in leasing, or write the copy for another page on my website. Then, when my clinic opened, I'd use that free time at work between patients to call our clinic patients back and book appointments.

In the beginning, I would be at the clinic seeing patients, doing all their paperwork, along with the admin work, while they were receiving their infusions. I figured that since I had to be there anyway, I might as well make the time productive instead of waiting around wasting time until they finished. A lot of times, patients didn't want to talk or be disturbed during their ketamine infusion therapy. So during their infusion, while I was sitting in the room monitoring them, I was also getting other tasks completed.

Now, I did have to make extra time in my schedule to get my clinic open, especially the several weeks leading into the opening. I did that by giving away shifts to colleagues, swapping shifts, and using some sick time. Those types of sacrifices are necessary to grow and build a better life. If it were easy, everybody would do it. And if everyone were doing it, it wouldn't be worth doing.

It's similar to going back to school. You wouldn't expect to go back and pursue another degree and not have to put in any extra time studying or attending lectures, right? The same thing applies when starting a practice. The biggest thing you can do to make it happen is to be more intentional with your time. Plan out your days and weeks. Adjust your schedule when needed. And stop wasting time watching TV, obsessing about the next game, or browsing the internet.

In the five-plus years that I've been a business owner and podcast host, I've met and interviewed hundreds of ultra-successful businessmen and women. Almost none of them waste their time watching excessive amounts of TV or scrolling social media feeds for hours at a time. Instead, they are putting those hours toward working on their business. They are reading books, listening to business podcasts, connecting with others, and attending events to grow their business.

If you want to be successful, you will have to make certain sacrifices in the beginning. And over time, you may realize that skipping that BBQ with the neighbor you don't even have much in common with anyway isn't even really a sacrifice.

Myth #6: I Won't Be Able to Find Any Patients

When I was getting started, I did some basic math calculations. I knew that the ketamine infusion therapy protocol recommended by *JAMA Psychiatry* was six infusions, so I only needed to help two patients with six infusions each to cover my monthly clinic operating expenses. But even with such a tiny number, I was still a little scared.

What I realized after opening is that patients in almost every part of the country were looking for these types of clinics, but often they had nowhere to turn and were forced to drive long distances for treatment. One of my students started her clinic after finding out that a family member was driving over five hours to get ketamine infusions.

When I was opening my clinic, I implemented just a few key pieces of marketing. As a result, I received dozens of calls and booked several patients before I even opened. The crazy thing for me was that there was another established ketamine clinic in my town, less than 10 minutes away. I thought for sure this competition was going to make it harder for me to get patients. Nope!

What I soon learned from my patients was that my competitor provided terrible customer service. His phone went unanswered, his available service times were not flexible, he didn't get back to his patients in a reasonable amount of time, and he was lacking in the compassion and empathy department. So a large number of his patients moved over to my practice once they saw me opening. The same thing happens all over the country.

I work with and stay in close contact with several dozen clinic owners, and many have told me that they have had very similar experiences with patients transferring into their practices. They opened a clinic across town from another practice that provided similar treatments and started getting patients simply because they answered their phones and provided a better, more compassionate patient experience.

In my case, over the first several months, my clinic saw rapid growth. I realized that my fears of not finding patients were completely unfounded. There are many people out there who have been wanting the services you can provide in a way that only you can provide them. They have just been waiting for a clinic to open close enough to them so they can conveniently receive the treatment they want and need.

Myth #7: Patients in My Area Won't Be Able to Afford It

Using our ketamine clinic as an example, when people hear that ketamine infusions aren't covered by insurance, the next thing out of their mouth is usually, "How do you get patients to pay for treatments then?" Trust me, I know they seem expensive when you're talking $350 to $750 per infusion. But stay with me here …

Mental health patients typically need six infusions, plus they return for boosters every four to six weeks. Chronic pain patients receive as many as 5 to 10 initial infusions, plus return for repeated booster infusions. So the total cost can be substantial for the patient. But assuming that no patient will ever invest that kind of money to get relief from their symptoms is just that: an assumption.

We often base assumptions on our own internal experiences, biases, and emotions that cause us to connect dots that aren't there. Contrary to what your initial thoughts may be, most patients can find the financial resources necessary to benefit from this treatment option.

Let's compare ketamine therapy to a massage. The price points are obviously different, but the overarching concept is the same. When I go to get a massage, I'll only go if it's in a dim, quiet room, with a soothing fragrance, and some peaceful music playing softly in the background. The masseuse must be a highly trained, licensed professional and have stellar reviews. The office must be immaculate and the service exceptional.

To have the type of experience I want, I know that I will probably pay three times more than if I were to get a massage in the back of a run-down industrial building or a strip mall in a not-so-nice part of town. And I'm okay with that.

Ketamine infusions, IV Hydration, and Aesthetics services are the same. Patients and their families want highly trained professionals to treat them. They want a beautiful spa-like practice with warm, smiling staff.

The majority of the middle class and upper middle class are willing to pay the out-of-pocket expense for treatment because it is an investment in their health, wellness, and self-confidence. The same holds true for any type of service you provide. One of the key reasons people choose one Med Spa over another isn't because the Botox is better at one location—it is because the *patient experience* is better.

If you're thinking of starting a practice that sells services at higher price points, you will want to do some market research to determine what services you should offer, what price points they should have, and what demographic you want to serve.

If you're in an area that's more rural and surrounded by a lower-income population, then opening a high-end clinic with the highest prices is probably not going to work for your market. Maybe the best option for your market is to keep prices lower so that you have a higher patient volume.

On the other hand, if you're thinking of opening your clinic in a larger city, you may want to create a high-end practice and provide "concierge services" to the ultra-wealthy. In every large city, there are moderate, high, and super-high income earners who won't bat an eye. They have disposable income and can see the value in the results you give them.

Once you determine what's possible in your area, the next choice you have to make is who you want to serve. Maybe you don't want to charge the patient at all. Maybe the best option for you is a non-profit practice with a focus on fundraising and providing a great deal of pro-bono work. Who you decide to serve and the prices you charge is a very personal decision and there's no wrong answer.

There are benefits and drawbacks to serving each segment of the population. At the end of the day, the people you choose to serve and the prices you choose to charge will be based on your passions and your vision.

Myth #8: Only a Physician Can Own a Clinic

We touched on this in the previous chapter, but I want to drive this home because it is so important to get rid of this misconception. The idea that you have to be a physician to own or open a clinic is simply not true in the majority of states. Even in the states that require a physician to own the medical side of the clinic, they often partner with administrators who run the entire operation. There are almost always legal workarounds in the few states where it may appear to be the case.

One of our students, Christy M., completely debunked this myth. Christy is a paramedic by training, living in California. California is one of those states that has some special hurdles to jump through for non-physicians. Due to its strict Corporate Practice of Medicine (CPOM) laws, it is actually one of the more difficult states for non-physicians to start a business that provides direct patient care. In that state, a physician has to own the clinic.

Christy found a workaround. She partnered with a trusted colleague who was a physician. Then she found a good lawyer to make sure she was structuring her practice in a way that was compliant with state laws.

It wasn't as easy as it could have been in other states, but it wasn't hard, either. First, she formed a corporation for the clinic, her physician partner was 100% owner of this corporation, and Christy sat as the Vice President. Then with the help of her attorney, she created a second corporation, a management services organization (MSO). The MSO handled all the administrative requirements of the clinic. And—*voila!*—she has a clinic and has complete control over the business side of the practice.

If Christy can do this in California, it can be accomplished in any state. The key is to ensure that state laws are followed in terms of who can own the clinic. The second key is to make sure you have a full understanding of the care that each type of clinician can provide given their license type and the state's scope of practice laws surrounding each license type.

For example, if you are a family nurse practitioner (FNP) or plan to hire one to work in the clinic, you need to understand that this type of professional can generally:

> "Diagnose, treat and manage acute and chronic diseases, while emphasizing health promotion and disease prevention. FNP practice includes, but is not limited to, assessing patients; ordering, performing, supervising and interpreting diagnostic and laboratory tests; making diagnoses; initiating and managing treatment, including prescribing medication and non-pharmacologic treatments; coordinating care; counseling; and educating patients, their families and their communities. FNPs can practice autonomously and, like other clinicians, coordinate with health care professionals to manage patients' health needs."[3]

---

[3] American Association of Nurse Practitioners, "Nurse Practitioners in Primary Care," May 2022, https://www.aanp.org/advocacy/advocacy-resource/position-statements/nurse-practitioners-in-primary-care.

The most critical part is understanding the state law and how the state law specifically describes what the FNP can do within their professional license, the state requirements around what they can do, and the state rules that detail the level of physician involvement, if any, that is required for an FNP to provide care or own a clinic that provides direct patient care.

Myth #9: I Won't Be Able to Find a Collaborating Physician or Provider

If you need a physician to be involved with your clinic, you will be happy to learn that there are dozens of companies that offer this service. A simple Google search for "collaborating physician," or variations on that search, will be fruitful.

This is a pretty low-key job for a collaborating or supervising physician. Typically they will be required to review and provide feedback on your protocols, review patient charts, and be available by phone in the event that you have to call them for a consultation.

They'll be getting paid well for what usually amounts to a handful of hours of work a month. Most states don't require the physician to be physically present, which makes this even more attractive for them. So you can open your search to include the entire state. There are plenty of physicians out there who would love to be a part of your clinic.

If you are a Registered Nurse (RN) or another type of licensed healthcare professional, you will need to hire or partner with a physician or another provider. You probably work closely with and already have great relationships with physicians and providers. So finding one to hire or partner with should be easier than you think.

As an RN, you will not be able to simply hire a "physician collaborator." This is a major mistake that has gotten many nurses in trouble with their licensing boards. The reason is that all patients must be evaluated by a physician or provider prior to treatment. The role of a physician collaborator is just to collaborate and provide recommendations; they don't evaluate patients and write orders for treatment plans. Instead, they collaborate with the providers working in the clinic.

As an RN, you must have a physician or provider working in your clinic. As we mentioned earlier in the book, a provider is an APRN, Physician, or PA, not an RN. RNs without advanced practice training and licensure are not authorized in any state to diagnose, order treatment plans that include medications, tests, or treatments that must be prescribed. So the simple solution for an RN is to approach a physician or provider they already know and then team up to create the clinic.

We typically see most clinics offering supervising or collaborating physicians between $1,000 and $1,500 a month as a flat fee. That can vary a little bit depending on region, but that's a very common range.

Take Action … and *Keep* Taking Action

So, you've worked on your mindset, addressed your fears, and shaken off limiting beliefs. You have also done some myth-busting. Great. Now what? The purpose of all of that is to get you to the point where you are ready to take action.

We'll discuss what actions to take in the following chapters. But right now, we need to address how to take action and how to *keep* taking action, in the face of the bumps that will come up in the road. And trust me, there will be bumps.

Starting and running a business is not a cakewalk. You're going to run into challenges that you have to overcome. All you need is to know the answer to one simple question: What is your "*Why*"?

Within nine months of my clinic opening, I was making more per month than I did as a full-time nurse anesthetist working in the hospital setting. Most importantly, I was helping patients and finally had control over my schedule.

I could plan a date night with my wife. I could go to the gym regularly. I started doing things that I actually enjoyed. I was able to hire enough staff so I didn't have to be at the clinic if I didn't want to. What I did with my time was completely up to me. I think more than anything else, *that's* what's made me the happiest—having freedom of choice.

I finally felt like I had found a worthwhile career that didn't completely consume my life. It took eight-plus years of stumbling through multiple degrees and jobs to get to that point, but I felt like I had finally done it.

Opening my own clinic ultimately allowed my wife and me to start a family of our own and move closer to my parents. I had always wanted to have kids, but prior to starting a clinic, it crushed me to think I wouldn't ever have the time to be the dad that I wanted to be. Now I can spend as much time with my kids as I want. I get the chance to see all of their firsts. That is everything to me. That's my "*Why*."

Why Your "Why" Is Important

Starting and running a business requires a great deal of learning and substantial effort. To be honest, it's not for everybody. If you lose sight of *why* you're actually doing what you're doing, then the odds of you giving up or throwing in the towel when you lose momentum are dramatically higher. But if you know your *why*, it will drive you to take action.

Knowing your *why* is the most important step you can take to ensure you remain on course while striving toward achieving your goals. When you know your *why*, you can always inspire yourself. Even during the most difficult times, you will find the strength to take the steps needed to keep moving forward.

When you ask people *why* they want to start a business, the answer you hear most often is "for the money." If you've said this before, I would challenge you to dig a little bit deeper.

Money is a superficial goal; it is never the true reason. Yes, it's the most obvious *why*, but it is not the most inspiring. It won't get you jumping out of bed excited when you know you have to do some things you simply don't feel like doing.

A person's *why* is their true purpose, cause, or belief that ultimately drives them to take action.

So *why* do you want the money? Is it for freedom from your job? So you can travel? To spend more time with your family? To have more control over your time? There is a simple process to discover your deep-down *why*. I highly encourage you to give this little method a try. You ask yourself "*Why?*" and then keep asking.

So you'd have a conversation with yourself that goes something like this:

> *Why do I want to start a business?*
>
> Because I want to make money.
>
> *Why do I want to make money?*
>
> I want to make money so that I can pay my mortgage. Duh.
>
> *Why do I want to pay my mortgage?*
>
> Obviously I want to pay my mortgage so I don't have the stress of missing payments and losing our house.
>
> *Why don't I want to lose my house?*
>
> Because I don't want my family living homeless.
>
> *Why don't I want my family to live homeless?*
>
> Because I love my family with my whole heart, and I don't want my spouse and children to worry about having a roof over their heads or food on the table. I want to keep the people I love safe and happy.

If you keep digging down like that until you get to a more vulnerable response, something will start really resonating with you. That is your *why*. Go back and remember that deep, vulnerable *why* when things are stressful and you feel like you don't want to do it anymore.

Your *why* will help you live with a sense of purpose. Having a purpose will compel you to take on challenges and stretch yourself further than you normally would. You'll be able to focus on the things that matter the most. Once you do that, the money follows. Ultimately, your *why* will help you live a happier, more fulfilled life.

Follow Your Dreams … Emphasis on the Word "Follow"

After determining your *why*, the next step you need to take is to dream. Dreaming is a sign that you have hope. It's a sign that you have some internal desire to change something for the better.

Dreams keep people feeling young; they keep them feeling vigorous and motivated. Dreams keep us all going. Christopher Reeve said, "So many of our dreams at first seem impossible, then they seem improbable, and then, when we summon the will, they soon become inevitable." Dreaming about what amazing things your future potentially holds is a valuable practice.

However, dreaming alone will not get you where you want to go. The overwhelming majority of people on this planet dream and just stop there. They end up living in la-la land because they don't actually do anything to bring their dreams to reality.

Taking action separates those who achieve greatness from those who swim in a crowded pool of average. A dream begins to work for you, and you can work for your dream, only when you transform it into a vision.

Dreams are blurry and lofty. They don't give you direction on how to get there. You must use your dream to construct your vision. Dreaming without a vision gives you false ambition. A vision develops as you create a clearer picture of your dream.

Visualization

Visualization is a super helpful practice to help you create your future. I used it quite a bit as I started out in business. Close your eyes and imagine what it would be like to wake up each day, fully in control of your time and destiny.

Imagine what it would be like never to have to work another holiday. Imagine having weekends off so you can make it to those date nights, football games, and dance recitals. Take a minute and think about everything you have wanted to do since starting in healthcare but couldn't because of the ridiculously demanding hours we all end up working.

Do you want to start a hobby? Or take more vacations? Have you wanted to spend more time with friends or loved ones? How about having more time to exercise or stretch? Or go on mission trips? If you could have even one or two of those things, how would it make a difference in the rest of your life?

With the right dream, the right vision, and a will to act, you are on the pathway to not only creating a successful business but also a more meaningful life.

SECTION TWO

Business Planning: Setting the Pace to Become a Healthcare Boss

TURNING YOUR DREAM INTO A VISION, THEN INTO YOUR REALITY

"It is never too late to be what you might have been."

—*George Eliot*

Now that you've gotten your mindset right, the next step is creating a business that aligns with your goals and vision for the future. Without proper planning, you set yourself up for failure. Planning helps to reduce risks and brings to light some common pitfalls you may not have even thought about. It also helps reduce expenses by cutting down on avoidable mistakes.

It is incredibly rewarding to own and operate a business that helps patients—or even saves lives. While I wasn't sure exactly what type of clinic I was going to open when I first started exploring my options, I knew it had to be one that really improved patients' quality of life. And I definitely wanted to start a clinic where I got to spend more time interacting with patients and their families.

Step one of the business planning process is envisioning your dream come to life. This helps to focus the mind. Remember that a dream is merely a wish until you take action on it. But a vision is a dream that can be acted upon. And a vision is the key to focusing on your dream. Once you have the images of what you want to create in your head, you can establish goals and work toward achieving them, thus bringing your dream into reality.

You absolutely must take the time to create the mental imagery of what it will be like day-to-day in your ideal dream clinic. This short exercise will help you envision your ideal practice. If you follow these steps with mental and emotional focus, it will give you a jump start on the process of building and running the business of your dreams:

> Find a quiet place to review the list below. Ask yourself the following questions, but be sure to pause and take a moment to really think about each one.

> Close your eyes. Take three slow deep breaths. Inhale for 3 seconds, exhale for 3 seconds, inhale for 3 seconds, exhale for 3 seconds, inhale for 3 seconds, exhale for 3 seconds.

Picture the answers to these questions coming alive in your mind:

- How big is my clinic?
- What colors do I see as I approach the building?
- What does the inside of my clinic look like?
- What kind of colors do I use? What's the decor? How does it make me feel?
- What does the waiting area look like?

- What do the rooms look like?
- For an IV therapy clinic, are there many infusion areas? Or only one open infusion room?
- Is there dim lighting, soothing music, and calming aromatherapy? What does that look like? How does it feel? How does it smell?
- What types of additional products and services are provided for my patients?
- Do I have multiple clinic locations?
- How many employees do I see when I walk into my practice? (Envision the smiles on their faces.)
- Do I work full-time or part-time?
- How do my patients feel after their treatments? (Picture them looking calm, relaxed, and happy.)
- How does that make me feel inside?
- Am I proud of what I've built? (Think about how much confidence you have gained and the person you've become through the process.)

Did you notice that you were envisioning something different with that final question? As you progress from novice to business owner, something will change. You will realize that when you reach your goal, you aren't even the same person.

You will gain a tremendous amount of savvy and confidence. You will have become more resilient and what I like to refer to as a "Healthcare Boss." And, yes, #healthcareboss is the hashtag for our community!

The questions suggested in the exercise above can begin to breathe life into your dream. Once you have worked through this a few times, you should have a crystal clear vision in place. Your next step is to create a vision board for yourself.

You can make your vision board powerful and effective by:

- Printing pictures of what your dream clinic will look like from the web or cutting out pictures from magazines.
- Including images that illustrate what you will *feel* like as a clinic owner. These pictures should elicit the *emotion* and the physical things that will be in your practice to help you daily.
- Pasting these images onto your vision board and hanging it someplace where you can see it daily.
- Spending at least five minutes a day looking at the board and envisioning your practice becoming your reality.

With a vision board in place, you want to actually have fun with it. Look at it and really *feel* what it will be like when you achieve that goal. (Notice I didn't say "if" you achieve your goal but "when.") This simple, crafty exercise will help to bring you more clarity and direction. When you feel it and see it as already yours, you are now in the right mindset to figure out next steps and more easily take action on them.

As an entrepreneur, the vision you have for the future of your business is what will drive you and your employees to success. Share your vision with your employees in every meeting. Without a shared vision regarding where the company should be headed, the business will wither.

For me, my vision was to create a tranquil ketamine infusion practice. We wanted to start by offering ketamine therapy first.

I had watched firsthand how the vicious cycle of depression can spiral someone into total despair. I found my *why*, which helped me form my vision for helping others suffering from mental health conditions. I pursued the vision, and in the end, my clinic ran just the way I dreamed it would.

Goal-Setting

Once you have dreamed of starting your own clinic, solidified it into a vision, and created a vision board to keep you emotionally inspired, the time for fearless action begins. Creating goals will force you to take action to make your dreams become reality.

There is a well-known method used to structure effective goals. It is an easy one to follow because it uses the acronym SMART. We always create SMART goals.

SMART goals must be Specific, Measurable, Achievable, Relevant, and Time-bound:

- **Specific** — For your goal to be specific, there should be as little ambiguity as possible in its formulation.
- **Measurable** — Attach metrics to your goal so you can measure your success and stay on track.
- **Achievable** — If you pick a goal that is impossible, you are defeating yourself before you even begin.
- **Relevant** — Your goal must help you achieve your vision, or you're just wasting your time. And speaking of time …
- **Time-bound** — Give yourself a deadline.

Let's take a look at how we could put this into action. Your major goal is to start a clinic, so we'll start there.

GOAL: Start a clinic.

Hmm, how SMART is that goal?

Now, let's try one that is specific, measurable, achievable, relevant, and time-bound ...

Open a self-pay IV clinic with four infusion chairs on October 1st that is booked two months ahead of opening.

Don't you think you'll be much more successful with the latter versus the former? In your SMART goal, there are specific attributes of the goal to aim for. Because you have metrics and a time constraint, you can tell when you're getting off track and how to get back on track. And this goal can be broken into smaller goals, which increases your chances of success.

A word on goals: make sure they are *your own* goals, not someone else's. The goals you choose have to inspire *you* and they must align with *your* vision. They have to matter to *you* or you won't do them.

Write your goals down. Put them somewhere you can see them every day. On your desk, your nightstand, the bathroom mirror ... whatever. Just have them in front of you all the time.

The "writing down" part of the goal seems like a rather simple task, right? Simple to the point where people don't even bother. You would be surprised at how few people actually write down goals, and how it hinders them from being able to achieve them.

Writing goals down and keeping them in front of you is a *really* important step in the planning process. The likelihood that you will achieve your dreams is substantially better if you get them down on paper. It is extremely difficult to stay on track without a written goal because a goal must be seen—and reviewed daily.

When you write your goals down, review them every day, and look at your vision board, after a while, you don't even have to think about your goals because they're so well-ingrained into your thought processes and your actions that they get imprinted into your subconscious.

Have I impressed upon you enough the importance of having written goals? Let's actually start creating the goals that will help you reach your dream and make your vision a reality. This means you move beyond just dreaming and visualizing to a point where you are setting goals and taking action to get to the end product.

Personal Considerations in Professional Goal Setting

Laurence J. Peter said, "If you don't know where you're going, you will probably end up somewhere else." Your professional goals should be dictated by your personal goals. First, you envision the life you want to lead. Then, as we discussed earlier, you only create goals that drive you in that direction.

Speaking of driving, how long do you want your commute to take? You'll be going to the clinic quite frequently, at least at the beginning. Do you want to drive an hour or more to work every day? Probably not. Use your personal goals and desires to influence your choice of the approximate location where you may want to start your practice.

How many hours a week do you want to work? How much money do you want to make? Who do you want to help, and how do you want to help them? Do you only want one location, or do you want to open multiple locations?

This isn't an all-inclusive list of questions, but it gives you an idea of personal factors that are going to come into play as you get ready to select your tentative or preliminary location. You won't have all the answers right away, and that's ok. You'll ask yourself a lot of essential questions that you won't be able to definitively answer until you analyze the market.

CHAPTER FIVE

MARKET RESEARCH AND ANALYSIS

"Give me five minutes to chop down a tree, and I will spend the first two and a half sharpening my ax."

—Unknown

Market research is another branch of your planning process. A general market analysis helps you predict how well you can expect to do in a given area. You draw your conclusions based on things such as location, population size, and demographics.

Those conclusions give you important information about the size of your market in terms of volume and value, demographics, and buying habits, as well as valuable insights about your competition. These will help you make a lot of big decisions such as location, pricing, and marketing. They will give you an idea about what buyer patterns might exist in that particular location and how saturated the market is. All of this leads to your ability to create a competitive advantage.

Through market analysis, you'll get a better understanding of the level of competition in an area, the economic nature of that environment, some barriers to entry, and some external forces like regulation and laws surrounding your type of practice. Market analysis helps you blend information about consumer behavior in that area with economic trends so that you can confirm and optimize your exact location.

The Different Aspects of Market Research

Your Ideal Client (Avatar)

You should have an idea of who your ideal customer is. Who do you want to serve? Know the type of clientele or patients your business is going to attract, as well as their characteristics. To do this, you'll need to develop your ideal customer or ideal patient avatar.

An avatar is a make-believe representation of your ideal client. Some businesses even give them a name, like Molly. Anytime they think of making a change in their business they ask, "Would Molly like this?"

This representation should be detailed, including things like:

- Molly's background
- Where Molly lives
- Her demographic information
- Her income
- Her diagnosis (if applicable) or why she is coming to see you
- What pain point she is trying to solve by coming to your practice

- What challenge(s) she might have faced when seeking out other practices or treatments
- Objections she might have to receiving treatment at your practice
- Her preferred way of consuming information

Certainly, the services that you decide to offer are going to influence your avatar. Just think about the people you want to help. What are they like? If it's a ketamine clinic, you're looking at someone who has tried other forms of treatment for depression or chronic pain and hasn't found any that work.

Some clinic owners may not want to deal with people with emotional or mental health issues. For others, the deal breaker might be low-income patients, while another clinic owner might love just that. There is no right or wrong, it's a matter of designing the perfect clinic *for you.*

Let's take KC for example. She is our co-founder and instructor of our IV Therapy Academy and she has chosen her avatar very wisely. In addition to her IV therapy practice, she also has a direct primary care (DPC) practice and her avatar is corporate benefit managers.

She sells her direct primary care service to small companies who offer her direct primary care services as a stand-alone benefit or who offer DPC benefits in addition to a high-deductible insurance plan. The value is affordable and accessible comprehensive primary care for their employees.

Many DPC clinics are going after one patient at a time, but she is scaling faster through employers and groups. She gives them something they can offer as an addition to a lower-cost insurance plan. It's essentially an unlimited primary care service for a monthly fee that she sells by going straight to company managers and getting 50–150 patients enrolled at a time. Now that is how you leverage scalability by choosing the best avatar.

Location

The first choice you're going to have to make about your clinic's location is which city you want to be in. That's usually pretty easy. Most people want to start a business near where they live, even if it's not in the exact same city. And again, you will choose an area that's within reasonable driving distance. These are the kinds of things you decide based on personal goals.

Remember, there are many things you won't be able to decide until you do the market research. This is especially true about exactly where you will put your clinic. The research you do will determine if your proposed location is in alignment with your ultimate goals, and if it's not, it will help you choose one that is.

The people you help and the kinds of services you offer will heavily influence your choices regarding location. For example, if your service model is an IV therapy practice, and you want it to attract walk-in patients, then maybe your location is going to be in an area with heavy foot traffic where patients can get quick service.

Clinics like this are very common in Vegas. Some casinos have IV therapy lounges where patients go in, get their IV hydration (aka hangover treatment), and they're off to the races again. Knowing your service model before picking a location is always a good idea.

Location research will provide you with quantitative and qualitative data regarding the market. Gathering the most relevant data will help you narrow down to a neighborhood or even a specific street address. We'll be talking more about the kind of data you want to be gathering and how to gather it later in the chapter.

Your Geographical Radius

This aspect of location has to do with looking at the catchment area of the geographical location around your clinic. Something I have found is that in almost every area, a majority of patients are willing to drive up to an hour to get to a practice.

Now, certainly, if you are a highly published or world-renowned expert, distance is no object, but for most clinicians, you'll be attracting patients within a reasonable driving distance. If you're starting in a rural location where there's no competition around, your catchment area could be a two-hour drive, or maybe even more.

When we were in Albuquerque, we were actually drawing patients from southern New Mexico, near the border of Texas. We had people who were driving four, five, and six hours to come to our practice for ketamine therapy. Some even flew in. That was several years ago though, and the competition around the country has increased. So, a catchment area of four hours away may not be the best bet in most markets today, but within a one-hour drive is very realistic.

Essentially, what you do is draw a radius of what you think is going to be the most reasonable catchment area for the location of your practice. There are a few online tools that can help you with that. They are designed to draw a radius around a center point or help you estimate the population in a very specific area. If you have an office location in mind, you can draw a several-mile radius, and the tool will help you calculate the approximate population within it.

Market Demographics

Researching things like the age, gender, income, and occupation of a given population is crucial to determining your market size. They hold important clues that help you predict consumer behavior.

If, for example, you are going to establish yourself in a neighborhood that has a lot of geriatric patients of below-average income, these people may not have a budget for discretionary spending and may be reliant solely on Medicare.

This type of information is going to help guide your decision on whether this is the best area for you. People with a similar demographic profile in the same location tend to have very similar purchasing patterns, so gathering demographic information can be very valuable.

Market Size

Market size is the number of people who are likely to buy your services within your service area. This is going to have a huge impact on what you expect the volume of patients coming to your practice will be. What percentage of the population does your ideal avatar make up? Basically, how many Mollys are there in your clinic's catchment area?

Population size is one of the most important things to look at in your analysis. The goals you have for your practice must align with the population size. If your goal is to run a practice full-time, you are likely not going to be able to do that in a town of 10,000 people. It would be incredibly difficult unless you have a very good strategy to bring in clients from a nearby city. If that volume doesn't align with your professional goals, then maybe you need to select a different location, or maybe you need to consider adding other services.

CHAPTER SIX

FINANCIAL PLANNING: KNOW YOUR NUMBERS

"The first $100,000 is a bitch, but you gotta do it. I don't care what you have to do—if it means walking everywhere and not eating anything that wasn't purchased with a coupon, find a way to get your hands on $100,000. After that, you can ease off the gas a little bit."

—Charlie Munger

If you haven't already decided on the services you will offer, you need that information before you can accurately figure out how much this will all cost and what you can predict your return on investment (ROI) will be.

This is where you start doing some financial calculations based on what products or services you are planning to offer. You will start listing your expenses. And you'll be putting together some estimates about the income you can expect. Once you have these numbers, you can start to generate some financial projections.

Financial projections are crucial decision-making tools for you as the business owner. If you will be seeking financing or talking to investors, financial projections will be mandatory. You'll need to have a good grasp of your numbers. This is both an art and a science.

If you're seeking any outside funding from venture capital, angel investors, or from banks, they're all going to want to see your financial projections. Financial projections are a "best guess" at what a business's revenue and expenses will look like in the future.

Obviously, you can't predict the future. Nevertheless, these guesses should be based on reasonable data. Everybody's projections are going to be different based on various factors that are unique to their particular business, location, avatar, services, and so on.

A word to the wise: it's a good idea to be conservative with your numbers. You don't want to take on too much risk.

Clearly, your projections will be influenced by your price point. A few things to consider when contemplating pricing are:

- The income demographics of your area
- Nearby clinics that are charging for similar services
- The type of customer you want to attract

In my opinion, setting your prices lower than your competition as a long term strategy is usually a terrible mistake. You are entering a race to the bottom—a race you do not want to win. Eventually, this type of decision is likely to drive you out of business. Instead, you could consider charging average or above-average prices for your area. This cost can be justifiable based on your focus on delivering exceptional service and value for the patients. This is a much better strategy for the long-term survival of your practice.

Patients associate quality with cost and if you are the Dollar General of practices, your clinic will earn a reputation as a cheap, low-quality practice that provides low-quality care. Avoid that kind of reputation by committing to not permanently setting your prices as the lowest in your area.

Estimating Income

The Income Statement

Estimating income is another aspect of the financial side of your business. As a business owner, one of the most important statements that you actually create on a monthly or even weekly basis is going to be your income statement. This is also known as your P&L (profit and loss) statement. This helps you get a good grasp of your numbers as a business owner.

You want to get really familiar with these statements and how to read them. But don't worry, they are pretty easy to read once you understand the basics.

The income statement is analogous to the vital signs of your business because it provides a snapshot of your business's revenue, expenses, and net income. It is typically data reported at least monthly.

Two common terms you will hear when it comes to income statements are "top line" and "bottom line." The top line is total revenue or gross revenue. It takes into account all the money brought into the practice through products or services sold. The bottom line is your net income, which is your gross revenue minus your expenses.

You work to increase your top line while finding creative ways to reduce your expenses. This is how you grow your business and your income.

Financial Projection Assumptions

Financial projections are based on a series of financial assumptions (as opposed to a pro forma, or financial forecast, which are based on historical numbers from your business). Do your research, find relevant information to give you useful data, and make your best guess.

Don't just take numbers from random findings and plug them into your financial projections. The information you'll find for Los Angeles won't apply to you if you're in Terre Haute. Different clinic owners in different locations will have different expenses, clientele, and price points. If you want accurate projections, you will have to put some effort into finding the most accurate numbers for your clinic.

Gross Revenue Projections

Your top line is completely dependent on your patient volume and your pricing. This is a reflection of a business's ability to sell goods and services, but not their ability to generate profit.

It bears repeating: while doing the numbers, I highly recommend making conservative estimates with your projections. If you get too lofty with your numbers, you could be setting yourself up for trouble. Always go conservative when you're estimating. Then you can be pleasantly surprised if and when you exceed them.

In our market, one thing I noticed was that in Albuquerque, there was a drop in patient volume in the late fall. It was around the holiday season (November, December). Another time we experienced a bit of slowdown was in the summer, when kids get out of school and families are taking their summer vacations.

These slowdowns may not happen in your market, or they may happen at different times. You want to keep these things in the back of your mind because revenue for every business is often cyclical or follows trends.

If there's a slow period for you one year, there's a very good chance you're going to have that same slow period the following year, as long as there weren't any sort of external events that caused the slowdown. If you know and understand your financial cycles and trends you can better manage expenses and therefore your cash flow during slower periods.

Estimating Operating (or Ongoing) Expenses

Estimating your typical operating costs involves calculating your anticipated recurring monthly expenses. We will do the overview here, but we'll go into more detail throughout the book.

Rent is a significant operating expense. The price will vary depending on your location and how big your clinic is. If you haven't found office space yet, use the space you came up with in your visualization and do some research. Look up how much your dream clinic will cost in the area you want to be in.

Depending on what kind of lease you have, you may have to pay utilities, janitor fees, common area maintenance, or a host of other expenses you may not have thought of. There are also a variety of different insurances that you will need to get. We will dive more into leases and the insurance you will need in a future chapter.

Your marketing will be part of your ongoing expenses. You'll be paying money for your website, any paid ads you run, brochures, and any mailers you print and send out. We'll also talk more about marketing in a later chapter.

Then there are supplies. You'll find that there are hundreds of little things you have to account for, but it's also a great exercise in visualization. If you mentally walk through the steps of the patient visit, including the care and the customer service components, you will have a much higher probability of creating an accurate list.

There are three main kinds of supplies: office, medical and pharmaceutical. Office supplies include things like paper, pens, clipboards or charts, staplers, hole punchers, printer ink or toner, light bulbs, and cleaning supplies.

Then it's time to think about medical supplies. That includes everything associated with providing medical treatment or services. For example, if your practice involves IV therapies, you're going to need IVs, IV tubing, syringes, gauze, bandages, medical tape, clear occlusive dressing, alcohol wipes, and more.

Lastly, there are pharmaceutical supplies, which include any of the medications you administer regularly as well as any emergency medications you may need to keep on hand.

We provide lists of office, medical, and pharmaceutical supplies in our training programs. You can learn more about them here:

jasonduprat.com/book

At some point, you will be hiring staff, which means labor expenses. Outsourcing legal and accounting is also an expense that is usually categorized as *professional services* on the P&L. If you are starting your clinic part-time, you might not want to hire a receptionist right off the bat.

Personally, I think it is a good idea to answer the phones yourself for the first several weeks, as things are growing. It will help you get a good grasp of the most common questions and you will also be able to better create processes for streamlining the patient experience and flow.

You will eventually be hiring either part-time or full-time medical, nursing, and/or support staff. That will cut back on the percentage of net profit you bring home, but it will increase the volume of patients that can be treated. It will also cut down the amount of time that you have to spend working in your practice.

Generally, labor expenses do tend to be one of the highest ongoing expenses for clinic owners, so you want to make sure you aren't overhiring staff. There is a balance to staffing that takes some time and experience to fine-tune.

Estimating Start-Up Expenses

Remember those goals and that vision we were talking about earlier? Your vision is a dream you can take action on, right? Well, here is where you start to take that action. That vision should be so clear that you can start totaling up its expenses as if it were already reality because that is what you're going to do now.

Let's jump back to your goals for a moment. If your goal is to completely replace and increase your current income, your practice will have to be relatively large and will require commensurate expenses. If your goal is to start a small, lean clinic and work up to a larger one, once you have optimized your operations and have some momentum, then the initial start-up costs will be less. Your numbers will also depend on the services you provide and the equipment that you need. How do you envision the interior? Any decorations or wall art, an aromatherapy diffuser, an audio system to play music—whatever you want to have when the doors open—all of that has to be accounted for.

Having a good estimate of your start-up expenses is critical in helping you get your practice started off on the right foot. Knowing these numbers goes a long way in ensuring you have enough capital to get your business going. If you do more hands-on work and less outsourcing of all the things that you need to get done to get started, a small practice can be started for as little as $20,000.

Let's say your goal is to triple or quadruple your six-figure income. In that case, you will need a larger practice that can treat a considerable volume of patients, and you will eventually need several providers to treat those patients. You will look for a more spacious office with more patient rooms and a break room. If you have several employees, they'll need a place to sit for lunch or to get a quick morning coffee, which means a break room and supplies—maybe a refrigerator and a Keurig too.

The good news about start-up expenses is that you can start purchasing some of the equipment while you're preparing to open. Most practices will take at least 90-120 days to open. During this time, you'll be getting everything planned, getting your lease signed, finding key team members, having an attorney review contracts, and the like.

This gives you an opportunity to spread some of your start-up expenses out over several months. You can use income that you're generating through work or your other business to start funding some of the start-up expenses. If you have investors or you have large sums of cash saved, then even better.

As you start to buy your equipment and spend money on things that you need to open, create an expense spreadsheet and keep all of your receipts in an envelope. You will scan those receipts before they fade out.

As soon as possible, you will want a business bank account and bookkeeping software because income and expenses can be more easily tracked and automated by linking your bank account with your bookkeeping software. Track all of your start-up expenses, and not just for tax purposes—it's super easy for runaway spending to take place if every dollar isn't tracked.

To stay within your start-up budget, you have to track your expenses, limit your wants, and invest only in your needs. There's always time down the road to reinvest capital back in your business.

Categories of Start-Up Expenses

In terms of start-up expenses, there are going to be different aspects of the clinic that you are going to categorize and lay out to estimate how much capital you will need specifically for starting up.

Construction and Build-Out Costs

After you've gone through and looked at your potential office location, you'll want to start factoring in some possibilities in terms of the physical changes you'll need around the clinic. Do you have to add a handwashing station? Do you need to add dividing walls? Are you going to build private patient rooms? What about restrooms or waiting rooms? Is there anything you need to do to comply with the Americans with Disabilities Act (ADA)? Questions like these are what you want to start thinking about and factoring into your start-up expense list.

We have created a free start-up cost calculator that is preloaded with the most common start-up expenses. You can get this tool at:

jasonduprat.com/book

Medical Equipment

There is a big difference between supplies and equipment. Supplies are anything you'll need to continuously order more of; they are also called consumables. Equipment includes the pieces of machinery you need to run your practice.

The type of practice you are opening will dictate the type of equipment you will need. Do your research. Cardiac monitors, for example, are one of the pieces of medical equipment that a ketamine clinic needs.

You'll also want a patient scale to get correct weight measurements. Patients are often inaccurate in estimating their weight, and if you are dosing on a per kg basis, having an accurate weight is vital.

You may also need thermometers and glucometers. In our ketamine clinic, we needed infusion pumps and automatic external defibrillators. Another piece of equipment you may need is a suction machine. Maybe you are starting a Med Spa. In that case, you may want a laser device. If you are offering platelet-rich plasma (PRP) or lab draws, you will need a centrifuge.

The list of equipment can be tiny or it could be very large and costly, it all depends on the type of services you plan to offer.

Licenses and Fees

Your start-up expenses are also going to include things like licenses and fees. All clinics will need a general business license from your city or county. If you're going to be administering controlled substances, you'll need a license from the Drug Enforcement Agency. You may need a pharmacy license or a state-controlled substance license.

Obviously, if you are a healthcare clinician, you will have a license that allows you to practice as a nurse, nurse practitioner, physician, or whatever your healthcare specialty is. You may also need a private practice license or a hazardous waste disposal license. Most of the exact requirements depend on your state's rules and regulations.

Marketing Expenses

There are some one-time costs with marketing and many ongoing ones. We touched briefly on the ongoing ones in the section on estimating operating costs. The one-time costs are things like the initial website build, branding, and design. We will discuss marketing in greater depth later in the book.

Office-Related Expenses

You're going to have an office, right? There are going to be costs associated with that. Some costs are ongoing, some will be one-time. The bulk of furniture and decor, for instance, will be a one-time expense. You will have to have a security deposit ready to go. Then there are costs such as the first and last months' rent. You may have small fees for initiating a new service like internet, electricity, gas, water, biohazardous waste, and garbage pickup.

All the lists of expenses mentioned above are not meant to represent a comprehensive list. Each situation is going to be a little different. You may find out that you do not need some of these, or maybe you'll need some things that aren't listed in this book. These items mentioned are intended to give you a good idea of what to start thinking about when considering your start-up expenses.

For a free start-up expense calculator head over to **jasonduprat.com/book** and register for one of our masterclasses. We have a free masterclasses on launching a ketamine clinic, IV therapy clinic, launching a Med Spa, and depending on when you are reading this book and visiting the page, possibly even more masterclasses that teach you how to launch and grow other healthcare businesses.

Bootstrapping

Bootstrapping is the process of using your existing resources to grow a company. It means taking on no investor debt to launch your practice. For most new clinic owners, there are typically a lot more pros than cons when it comes to bootstrapping.

Certainly one of its major cons would be that the amount of funding available for the business is going to be dictated by your own personal financial situation. If you're a healthcare professional, then you're likely already starting with above-average income, depending on your license type, maybe even far-above-average income, but that doesn't necessarily mean you have large amounts of cash reserves.

I know firsthand that many healthcare professionals are saddled with mountains of student loan debt for several years after graduating. I had over $130,000 in student loan debt after finishing my nurse anesthesiology program and was working overtime to pay extra on my loan bill, which was larger than my mortgage.

You may want to keep your full-time job as you're getting things off the ground. You may need the income from your full-time job to fund your start-up. Or you may need to wait a year or two and get your personal finances in order first. I lived very frugally for years and followed the snowball method taught by Dave Ramsey to reduce my debt and increase my savings.

When you're the only person putting all the capital into your business, you have more to lose because it's all your money. But everything in business is a risk/reward ratio, so if you have a bit more risk, you're going to have a higher potential return on the backend.

One pro of bootstrapping and starting small is that you can start a practice for as little as $20,000. It simply takes a focus on starting lean, but *never* skimp out on investing in an attorney and hiring an accountant. I'll keep saying it throughout this book because they are very important, yet many skip this step to save some money. Hopefully, it'll stay with you.

Bootstrapping does *not* mean taking shortcuts in order to cut costs. Shortcuts like these will increase your risk exposure. It is *not* worth "saving the money" that it would cost to hire professionals. They can save you from a world of hurt and mistakes.

Do not cut corners on legal or accounting. Investing in professional advice is critically important, especially legal advice. Just one missing sentence or even a single word from an employment contract or a patient consent form can mean the difference between winning and losing a legal dispute.

One tiny misinterpretation or assumption you might make related to your scope of practice could cost you your license. Failing to properly file a state or federal tax document or state unemployment record could cost you hundreds or thousands in penalties and late fees. You need to set aside several thousand dollars for legal and accounting advice upfront and you also want to budget those service costs into your ongoing expenses.

One of the best ways to bootstrap your way to success is to start with a small location and enter into a short-term lease. Consider getting a lease that's a year or two at the most. Sometimes when the economy is booming, that can be hard to find, but it's hands down the best way to do it.

Then, as soon as you start to outgrow that small practice, within a year or two, you can very easily move to a different location that is larger and can support your growth. By doing it this way, you just reduced your financial risk.

Jumping into an oversized clinic and costly lease without an established patient base is a common mistake among new clinic owners. It's hard to be profitable quickly if you have a lot of debt or if you carry ongoing expenses that are out of proportion to the volume of patients you are helping. For most clinicians, success is all about starting small and on a budget.

Don't go crazy on things like office decor. You can still have an attractive practice that is affordable. In my case, I shopped around online until I found the most beautiful reception desk. It was gorgeous and one of only a few things I purchased new. It happened to be the most expensive item I invested in for the start-up. The reception area is the first thing patients see when they walk in, so I felt strongly that it needs to look great. It still only cost me $1,000.

Sometimes buying used is the only way to get a deal, but if you shop around, deals can be found on new items as well. Get resourceful and look for ways to save money that do *not* increase your risks or liabilities.

Ideally, you should have several months of start-up expenses, living expenses, and an emergency fund set aside. In my opinion, you should not be taking out huge loans unless you have business experience or an established patient base that you can bring from another location. On that note, be very careful to read any non-compete or non-solicitation agreements you may have signed prior to bringing patients from another work location.

There's nothing wrong with taking out a small loan, but putting hundreds of thousands of dollars on your credit cards or on a new business line of credit is generally not a good idea and greatly increases your risk and your time to profitability.

Minimizing Your Start-Up Expenses

There are a few other ways to minimize your start-up costs. Probably the best way is to put in a bit of sweat equity. For example, say you order some cabinetry. You, your spouse, your business partner, or your kids can assemble them. If the walls need a coat of paint or two, do that yourself.

You could apply the same concept in building a website. There are plenty of online tutorials on how to go about it. We even built a tutorial into all of our clinic start-up training programs. It's actually simple. Anybody who can use Microsoft Word can build their own website to get started because understanding code is no longer required.

Yup, you read that right, you don't have to write a single line of code to build a website these days, it's all drag-and-drop interfaces now. You just need to understand a few simple concepts to get your clinic website to show up on the first page of Google, which we also teach in our training programs.

You should also be careful with the amount of supplies that you initially order. Only order your first two or three weeks of supplies. Then gradually build your stockpile of medical supplies as time goes on and when income rolls in. Look into medical supply distributors and wholesalers.

Now that we have three training academies and thousands of students, we were able to negotiate a deal with one of the largest distributors in the US, which saves our students 10% to 14% on their medical supply orders. Other organizations or associations may be able to secure discounts that you can also leverage.

Ideally, you should have your business bank account set up before you start purchasing anything for your business. If you set up your account early, you can make your initial deposits of start-up capital into the business account, then use that business bank account to make all your clinic-related purchases. That's going to make things very simple to track when you reach the end of year one, and you have to submit all of your information to your accountant to do your taxes.

Take my advice on this one, set your business up early and have that business bank account ready to go as soon as possible. This will make your bookkeeping and expense tracking a breeze.

Once your business account is open, NEVER, I repeat NEVER pay business expenses from your personal account and NEVER pay personal expenses with your business account. This creates a major liability issue that is outside the scope of this book, but your attorney can fill you in on it, just ask about *piercing the corporate veil.*

Navigating Your Funding Options

Now that we've talked about bootstrapping your clinic launch with the resources you have available to you, there are several other avenues that you can take to fund your practice.

Outsourcing (Informal Investors)

If you decide not to completely fund the practice yourself, there are other ways you can gather the capital you need. You can look for informal investors. This would include friends and family, or maybe even close colleagues you know well. Create a pitch deck, or some sort of document, to help walk you through a presentation. Manage their expectations as far as what kind of return they should expect on any capital that they provide you.

Even if your informal investors are friends or family, you really want to keep things professional. This will set the stage for what they can expect from you in the future. You may need to go back to these individuals later for a second round of investment capital for the next phase of growth. You will want to maintain a professional and collaborative attitude from day one.

I don't typically like this option because this is a business, and not everyone who tries will actually succeed. There will always be some clinics that end up closing their doors for a wide variety of reasons.

If things do not go as anticipated and you can't afford to pay the person back down the road, there's a good chance that your relationship will be damaged. For that reason, this isn't an arrangement to be jumped into lightly.

Bank Business Loans

Bank loans are another funding option, but the application process can be lengthy. Most banks prefer to work with established businesses. There are some, however, that will work with new businesses.

The pros, in this case, are that you get to still retain complete control of your business. But, as with any loan, you also generate a debt obligation to the lender. Interest rates also tend to be lower and terms are typically longer compared to personal loans.

New businesses usually require good personal credit. Unless you have an established business with a solid track record of profitability, banks will typically require a personal guarantee, meaning if the business fails, you are still personally obligated to repay the bank with personal funds.

Just like most loans, if you fail to repay them, the bank can take you to court, and a judge could force the sale of personal assets to fund the repayment of a loan that is in default.

Small Business Administration Loans

Another option is a small business administration (SBA) loan. They're still a type of bank loan, but they're partially secured by the government. This means that the government is agreeing to pay back a portion of the loan balance in the event your business could not meet its obligation to pay back the loan.

Since the government will guarantee that the bank will get at least a certain percentage of that loan back, this reduces the risk to the bank, which makes them more eager to loan to new and small businesses at a more affordable interest rate.

These types of loans are often lower-interest, longer-term, and a bit more flexible, though they still require good credit. Oftentimes, these loan types are actually better for existing businesses or to purchase an existing business.

For start-ups, they like to see an owner with a solid track record of business success because funding for a new business is riskier than, say, purchasing a business that's been in operation for years and has a decade-long track record of generating positive income. You can learn more about these loan options at sba.gov.

Personal Loans

Personal loans could also serve as a funding option, depending on the situation people find themselves in. The application process is usually fast, but the interest is usually higher and the loan term is often shorter when compared to a business loan.

In this case, depending on the size of the loan, you may have to put up collateral like your home, vehicles, or other valuables, and they can be repossessed if you do not make payments, so there tends to be a higher risk.

Credit Cards

Do not use credit cards for borrowing large amounts of capital. I know there are those clickbait headlines where some get-rich-quick training says otherwise. You might even see legitimate stories of somebody who's used a credit card to invest in an initial business and got lucky. Those cases are few and far between.

If you rack up debt on a credit card, it's extremely hard to get out from underneath it because the interest rates are so high and the repayment terms are generally non-negotiable.

Also, don't forget you are personally liable for any credit card debt you accrue. This includes nearly all business credit cards. Don't believe me? If they ask for personal information—your social security number, for example—they are running your personal credit report.

Read the fine print on any business credit card application, and you will find that you are personally responsible for payments if your business can't make them, which is why they are asking you for your personal information in addition to your business's.

Venture Capital

Unless you have some extremely unique ideas or some really amazing connections and lots of business experience, then you can probably rule out venture capital pretty quickly. Most venture capital investors are firms or funds that focus on investing in businesses with the potential to rapidly grow, serve the masses, and produce massive returns. In most cases, you need to have some really unique angle and a major growth strategy for them to invest. In general, a small practice is not going to qualify for venture capital, but if you did, you will also be trading equity for that capital.

Also, sometimes you are required to give these venture capitalists a decision-making role in the business because they want to make sure that they increase the odds of it being successful. In other cases, they want to have a say in making sure that the business has the best leaders in place to take it to the next level.

Angel Investors

Angel investors can also serve as a source of funding. Typically, these are high-net-worth investors who invest capital and their expertise for equity. There are online platforms and associations where you might want to seek out some angel investors, a simple Google search will yield many results.

Shark Tank is a pretty good example of how angel investing works. These investors will put up capital in exchange for equity. Many will also add value to the business by providing access to their expertise, their connections, and other resources to help the business grow.

Crowdfunding

Lastly, there is the crowdfunding option, and this option comes in different forms. One is a rewards-based type of funding source. In this case, you will typically provide something in return for somebody investing in your business.

Let's use the example of a start-up eco-clothing line. For a $5 donation, they'll send you some socks. A $25 donation will get you a cap. Asking for donations gives you access to cheap money, and the pro is you don't have to give away equity. The con is that not only do you have to provide a tangible reward but you also have to hit your funding target—or you don't get any money at all.

Typically, the funding that comes in, is through thousands of small donations, versus big capital investments, so if you don't hit your funding target, it could potentially be a huge waste of time.

Another crowdfunding option is equity-based crowdfunding. This is basically exchanging capital for a percentage of equity in your company or for shares. The pro of this is that you can get funding from angel investors who make a smaller investment than, say, going to just a single angel investor.

Start Smart

Starting a medical practice can be a substantial investment, but expenses and risk can be reduced by bootstrapping and starting small. It is important to always invest in legal and accounting advice and to budget for these services in ongoing expenses. Starting with a small location, a short-term lease, and planning on moving to a larger location as the practice grows are great ways to save money and reduce risk.

In general, it is wise to avoid taking out large loans or putting significant amounts of debt on credit cards. Instead, you can minimize expenses by putting in some sweat equity. If you are mindful of expenses and assess risks associated with your cost-saving measures, you will greatly increase your odds of success.

CHAPTER SEVEN

DESIGNING YOUR PRACTICE FOR JAW-DROPPING SUCCESS

"He who said money can't buy happiness hasn't given enough away."

—*Unknown*

The next thing you want to start planning is how to structure the business itself with the information you have gathered. Look at the business from a long-term point of view. How do you structure it to last? How do you make it stand out? What information is out there that you can leverage to put you ahead in your market?

There is a lot of analysis that goes into answering these questions. There are actually several different kinds of analyses that you will be performing, so let's dive in and talk about them.

Competitive Analysis

One of the best ways to learn, is to learn from others who have achieved what you want to achieve. Study the most successful practices in your state and study your top-performing competitors. Find out what they offer, how they offer it, and what their customers are saying about their service.

Analyzing your competition is going to help you figure out a competitive edge and a strategy to differentiate your practice. It's also going to help you determine the level of market saturation. You'll get a good idea of how many locations providing similar services are in your vicinity.

The first step to conducting a competitive analysis is to search the geographical area where you're tentatively planning to start your practice. Some choose to draw a few-mile radius around the potential location, while others will encircle everything within an hour's drive. However you decide to do it, find all the competitors in that area.

Don't get overly focused on the number of competitors, though. If you see there are several competitors, it is silly to throw up your hands and give up this early in the analysis process. The point of analyzing the competition is to find out what they're doing well and implement something similar. More importantly, it's to formulate a plan to have your clinic dominate in areas where the competition falls short. That's how you can differentiate yourself and your clinic.

Let's go back to our ketamine clinic example. Maybe your competitor uses ketamine to treat mood disorders but doesn't also offer psychotherapy or in-house psychiatry services but you do. Maybe they are way overpriced or maybe they are way underpriced. They might be in a bad location, or their practice isn't that nice inside or their customer service is terrible. Maybe they don't invest in marketing and struggle to get patients.

Competitive analysis is about trying to figure out where your practice can fit in. If you're running your practice well, and you're offering high-quality care and services that other clinics aren't offering, you are bound to excel.

It could be something as simple as being able to text with patients. You would not believe how many clinics don't have texting capability, don't answer their phones, or fail to call potential patients back. It's crazy. They're running a business. They have nobody to remind patients about their upcoming appointments, or no system to track and reschedule no-shows. Simple omissions like these are what you can easily take advantage of.

Next, take a look at the different directories that are out there. Search them to get a better understanding of competitors in your area. Make sure you're not leaving any clinic off of your list. If you get sloppy and miss a main competitor, it could make the difference between success and failure.

Once you've created your list of competitors, gather even more intelligence on them. Further analyze each one. Look at their appointment booking process. You or a friend can call them pretending you're a patient and book an appointment. You can always call back and cancel later. Check out how streamlined their process is—do they respond right away?

We had a competing clinic in our city that did a horrendous job of being responsive to patients or those with inquiries. They didn't ever call people back. So many of their patients left them to come to us for something so simple. It boggles my mind. *They didn't call people back and they didn't answer their phones.* Something like that can be used to your strategic advantage when you're starting your practice.

You also want to analyze how good their customer service is, not only on the phone but also via their email and text etiquette. Can a customer email them and ask a question? Do they actually respond? Do they respond in a polite fashion, or are their responses short and sort of rude? What's the response in person if you were to go there and ask some questions or ask for a consultation?

Look at their marketing campaigns. Do they market on social media? Do they even have social media accounts? Do they use paid ads? Do they send out email marketing? Do they have print marketing?

I always recommend that you scope out all your closest competitors in person. Go look at their practice. Take note of things you see as you approach the building and things you see inside. Go sit in their parking lot at different times of the day.

Most business owners skip steps like these because they feel awkward, but it is important observational research. Do they have enough parking? Is the parking lot well-lit? Is it clean? What's the overall appearance of the exterior of the building? Do you walk directly into their office when you arrive at their location? Or do you have to hunt your way through a massive office building, getting lost looking for signs?

Look at other types of services they offer. Check out their pricing and their payment options. All this intel you're gathering can be used to help you figure out how you're going to do things differently and better.

Go to Google, Facebook, the Better Business Bureau, and Yelp and read their reviews to see how they've been treating their patients. Note that reviews tend to be a little bit biased because most people who have a good-to-average experience are probably not going to take the time to pull out their phone and leave a Google review. But the people who are angry and feel like they had a terrible experience will certainly do that.

Keep in mind that some clinics will pay overseas Google review companies who unethically leave hundreds, if not thousands, of fake reviews. This is against Google's terms of service, and they will eventually get caught and will be banned from Google. Don't be tempted to use this short-sighted strategy! The long-term risk is not worth the short-term gain. Plus, you risk losing your money when working with unethical service providers like these.

Look to see if your competitors have received any awards or regular media attention. Do they have any notable industry leaders on their team? Is there a provider who's constantly being interviewed as a leading expert? All those are going to be factors you want to take a look at.

Find out roughly how much market share they have. What are they doing well? And what is that thing you think you might be able to do better—or have a different angle on? What are they doing poorly? What about their product or service is not meeting the needs of the patients?

Try to answer these questions about each competitor. These are all going to help you develop your business plan. When you have finished doing all this analysis on your competitors, don't forget to apply your analysis to the future business that you are setting up.

Environmental Analysis

Environmental analysis involves gathering information related to external factors that can impact your business. Look at the political environment: what rules or policies are governing your specific location? Each municipality has different rules. These rules may be more strict or more lenient than other municipalities.

Find out what the rules are in your anticipated location. Pay particularly close attention to Corporate Practice of Medicine (CPOM) laws and to Scope of Practice Regulations. How are the overall economics doing in that region? And then as a whole, how are the macroeconomics going in the entire nation, or even in the entire world? Those are important things to look at socioeconomically.

What other external changes might come into play? Is a new technological advancement impacting the delivery of your product or service? Stay abreast of these factors so you can respond to any changes. There could certainly be opportunities or threats to your practice as these external factors evolve.

SWOT Analysis

SWOT is a common business acronym that stands for Strengths, Weaknesses, Opportunities, and Threats. You'll want to do a

SWOT analysis using all the intel you've gathered so far, including the plans for your future practice. Analyze all of the strengths, weaknesses, opportunities, and threats in terms of starting and running your business.

Strengths

What will you excel at? What will set you apart from your competition? This could be your customer service, your personal reputation as an expert, a better technology or technique, the brand of product you use, the superior quality of your self-branded supplement, or anything else that you do better than the other clinics in your market.

Weaknesses

What are some of the weaknesses that your future practice might have? Maybe you're a first-time business owner with no marketing knowledge or experience. That might lead to launching a weak marketing campaign. Or maybe you're starting with extremely limited funds. You might need to offer fewer services until you have the capital to invest in training or the equipment needed to provide additional services.

Granted, your personal and business weaknesses are not fun to think about. I get it. But self-awareness is fundamental to planning your practice and to your future success.

Opportunities

Now, look at all the opportunities that exist for your practice. How can you leverage the gaps that are in your existing marketplace to the advantage of the practice? Can you offer better treatment hours? Can you offer better customer service by leveraging software with automation that improves the patient experience?

What about in-home service? Can you offer a more upscale clinic setting compared to others, or maybe you want to go the opposite route but also have a lower price? Look for gaps in the market and think about how you can fill them. If you do this well, you will have a thriving clinic.

Threats

What threats does the competition pose? Do they seem to have a large number of influential friends or business associates? Are they backed by angel investors or have extensive access to capital? Are they so well-established as a market leader that it's going to be hard to take market share from them? Are they the type of competitor that goes around and buys up all the existing practices?

Pending regulatory changes could also be a potential threat. You always want to have any new laws or new regulations on your radar. Large employers moving out of an area could mean population decreases and reductions in local income. Those warning signs could potentially tell you that maybe that's not the best location to get started.

Use all the information from your SWOT analysis to design a practice that has the best chance of success. Keep your personal and professional goals in the back of your mind and keep your emotions out of it.

Depending on what you find, you may consider altering your plan. It could turn out that the business doesn't actually line up with your goals. You may even decide that this is not the right business for you. These are the things you want to know before you make major capital investments.

Your Team

Once you've done all the analyses and have decided it's a go, it's time to start putting together your team. These are the people who will be playing a crucial role in getting your clinic up and running.

Hold off hiring non-critical roles until you have to. There are probably going to be some people you *must* have in place before you start. You want them to be the best people you can find. The groundwork they lay will determine the potential for growth and the sustainability of the business for years to come.

Accountant

Don't settle for a mediocre accountant. Get someone who knows what they're doing and who specializes in working with health-care professionals. I have seen people who were so concerned about saving every last penny when they were getting started that they didn't even bother to find an accountant. They try to do everything themselves. That's probably one of the biggest mistakes you can make.

If you don't have a thorough understanding of tax write-offs, how to properly allocate the start-up expenses, what forms to file and when, or any of a number of essential accounting items, you're going to have to fix a lot of finance and accounting mistakes down the road. It's better to just prevent them from happening.

When it comes to accounting, it benefits you to have some basic knowledge of tax planning and bookkeeping. It is super important to think about taxes way before it's time to file. This will help you reduce your tax liability.

There are hundreds of thousands of business owners in the US who legally pay little or no taxes. You can do that too. It's not that they're cheating the system; the tax laws are set up to provide advantages to business owners. A good accountant understands how tax laws work.

Tax codes exist to stimulate the economy and promote the prosperity of our country and its citizens. Tax breaks tell you what the government wants people to invest in. They want people to invest in business, real estate, energy, and agriculture. Taking advantage of the tax breaks will help businesses, like yours, to thrive in the long run. And thriving businesses are one of the key components of a healthy economy.

It's important to grasp the underlying principles here. You don't have to become an expert in tax law, but understanding the concepts behind it helps you understand how it impacts your bottom line. It will also help you in finding accountants and tax advisors that have the knowledge and background to help you with proper tax planning.

One of the really good books that I read about tax laws was *Tax-Free Wealth* by Tom Wheelwright, Robert Kiyosaki's accountant. It's a great book that shows you the ins and outs of how and where it's possible to save money on taxes. I had the pleasure of having Tom and some other great accounting and tax experts on my podcast. You can listen to the podcast here:

jasonduprat.com/listen

Finding a skilled accountant is critical. One common question I get is, "Should I only consider hiring a Certified Public Accountant (CPA), or will an accountant without that certification do just as well?" In my opinion, professional experience and track record always trump additional degrees and certifications.

CPAs are accountants that have passed an exam and have demonstrated their level of knowledge through that exam and certification. They are authorized to provide a couple of additional services that a non-CPA can't. First, they can represent a client in front of the IRS. And second, they can prepare financial reports for the Securities and Exchange Commission. Having a CPA may be beneficial, but it doesn't mean they are better. These extra capabilities that a CPA certification allows for don't directly provide a small business owner with any advantage.

A good accountant isn't someone who just prepares your tax returns. The good ones do way more than that—they save you money in taxes and help reduce your risk of getting audits. On top of that, a really good accountant can help you analyze and make good financial business decisions.

It's really important to have a dynamic working relationship with your accountant. They should be available for consultation anytime you make big purchases or sales. A good accountant can also help you understand various retirement accounts that you might qualify for and help guide you in choosing the best one to open for your specific situation. Or, at the very least, be able to refer you to a retirement account specialist.

Your bookkeeper or accountant will record your spending and reconcile any money coming in or going out by analyzing your bank statements. I think it's a very smart idea to use a bookkeeping software to simplify the process. You want to be on top of your business' finances.

Bookkeeping software like QuickBooks Online helps you track your accounts and expenses. Most bookkeeping software will connect to your business bank account and can automatically categorize recurring transactions and run reports for P&Ls, balance sheets, and statements of cash flow. They make it easier to keep your eye on your company's bottom line and can make tax preparation go much more smoothly.

When you hire an accountant, make sure to let them know if the attorney who set up your corporation applied for an employer identification number (EIN) for you. If they have not, then your accountant can do it or you can apply for yourself on the IRS website.

You will be assigned a number immediately, and within a couple of weeks, you get the official letter in the mail. Your EIN is essentially the social security number for your business. It is a nine-digit number assigned by the IRS used to identify the tax accounts of employers and businesses. Keep a copy handy, you're going to need it to open up a business bank account and certain retirement accounts.

Attorney

I nearly got into some serious scope of practice trouble when I first opened my clinic. I had received some bad advice from the attorney who was writing my clinic's contracts for freelance providers. Scope of practice issues are serious and they can potentially result in losing your ability to practice.

As I mentioned earlier in the book, there was a competitor nearby who ran his practice terribly. When we opened, many of his patients left his practice and became patients of mine. Naturally, he wasn't happy about that, so in a desperate attempt to get his patients back, he reported me and my clinic.

I had done hours of regulatory research and received informal advice from my contract attorney. This attorney also happened to work for the anesthesia group I worked for. In fact, one of the partners in this successful group referred me to this attorney, so I trusted him. When this attorney told me he believed my practice model was compliant, I didn't think anything else of it.

Well, this frustrated competitor spotted an area where he thought I was out of compliance and filed a complaint with the state's Board of Nursing. I still remember this day like it was yesterday.

Long story short, I received a hand-delivered letter from two Board of Nursing investigators flashing badges who had come to notify me of this competitor's allegation and I was completely shocked. I had no idea that there was even a remote possibility that I was out of compliance.

Since I wasn't able to get an appointment with another attorney who specialized in scope of practice issues for a few weeks, I had to immediately make changes to the structure of my practice just in case.

Several weeks later, I learned that I was, indeed, operating out of compliance. As a result of this huge mistake, I spent over $10,000 on attorney fees to respond to the complaint and ended up suffering months of stress and many sleepless nights.

That was a mistake I could have avoided if I had hired a specialized attorney who actually knew the state's laws regarding the establishment of an independent clinic and nurse anesthetist scope of practice regulations. It was also the event where I learned that not all attorneys are created equal. Just because an attorney can write contracts for healthcare workers, it doesn't guarantee they know anything about scope of practice regulations.

I simply didn't know better at the time. I had no experience working with attorneys, and I was lacking fundamental knowledge about the practice of law and how to properly engage or vet an attorney. I also didn't formally retain him to provide advice specifically related to scope of practice. Had I retained him for his advice on how I structured my practice, I could have had some recourse related to his erroneous assessment.

Experience and specialization in scope of practice regulations and clinic compliance are vital when it comes to hiring an attorney to provide guidance on how to structure your clinic based on the services that can be performed by various license types.

I highly encourage you to read your state's scope of practice rules and regulations and make the investment upfront to hire a *specialized* attorney who can help guide you through any state-specific legal requirements and help you determine what, if any, scope of practice limitations you may have to overcome in your state.

A good attorney or attorneys will help you structure your business, protect personal assets, file the right paperwork, create and review consents, and dozens of other little things that you will probably overlook because you don't know they're there. Don't fall victim to an attorney who claims to be able to handle *all* your legal needs. A jack of all trades is a master of none. Hire a specialist for each legal question or challenge you encounter.

Most states have an option for attorneys to get board-certified in various specialties. It's not mandatory that you have a board-certified attorney. Don't be fooled by a board certification either. This certification doesn't mean they have experience helping clinics get started. If you're launching a small practice, you want to work with an attorney who has a lot of experience working with small medical practices, ideally with clinicians that have the same type of license you have.

A board-certified healthcare attorney who only works for large corporate entities is probably not the right attorney for you. They may not have any idea what the rules and regulations are for a small private practice if they specialize in corporate healthcare law.

Just as in the case of accountants, make sure that the attorney's experience is very similar to your exact situation. If you're an

APRN, make sure they have experience working with APRNs who have started practices. If you're a physician, you want to know if they've helped other physicians start-up practices and maintain compliance. Don't pay somebody $350–$600+ an hour to do research and "figure it out" when you could find somebody who already has experience in that area.

Payroll Company

Attempting DIY payroll is generally not something a new business owner should be tackling. Find a payroll company and have them do it for you. The cost is pretty minimal and they will help you manage direct deposits, automatic withholding of payroll taxes, employee benefits, payments for unemployment insurance, worker's compensation, and sending out year-end W-2s or 1099s. They can customize your payroll reports and will often-times include some HR services for a small charge to help you onboard new contractors or employees.

Every employee will need to have a W-4 completed before you pay them so that the proper amount of payroll tax is withheld. They will also have to fill out an I-9, and you will attest that you verified the documents needed to prove that they're legally able to work in the US. For contractors, you have to have them complete W-9s; keep them filed in your records so that you can report your 1099s with the IRS.

There is a lot that goes into this, and hiring a payroll company makes it so much easier. Typically, these services will have tiers or different plans that you can enroll in. If you want only the basics as you're starting out, you can get a package that doesn't include any HR, benefits management, or any other bells and whistles. Then, you can upgrade as your practice grows.

Clinical Staff

Most clinic owners are licensed healthcare professionals who begin working as the clinic's primary clinician and then hire other clinicians as volume increases. As your business grows, consider which type of professionals can provide various aspects of the services you will be offering. This is based on what the regulations in your state dictate.

There are a variety of ways to structure your clinic staffing. The most important aspect of determining your staffing structure will be the laws of the state in which you practice. Check with your state's Medical Board, Board of Nursing, Board of Pharmacy, Department of Health, and other state boards to get a firm understanding of the scope of practice and state regulations.

Another important thing to consider is patient safety. It is highly advisable to have a provider on-site who is capable of performing advanced patient assessments and ordering any out-of-the-ordinary or emergency treatments that may be necessary. The staff in your clinic must be able to handle any potential emergency that could arise—as rare as those cases may be. Some states actually mandate that a provider be in the clinic or at least available for teleconsult when a patient is in the clinic, so it is critical to know what the rules and regulations are in your state.

When hiring a provider for your clinic, you might come across people who want to be more than just your W-2 employee. I've seen a lot of new clinic owners get taken advantage of because the person they hired said that they wanted to be an owner, or they wanted to be given a percentage of the business in exchange for being the provider.

If you want to do a profit-share with your provider or supervising physician, you absolutely can. (Do not confuse this with a kick-back for a referral as those are very different things.) I actually recommend offering profit shares or bonuses *after* they have proven their loyalty and commitment to helping your business succeed. It's a great way to get key employees to stick around longer.

Keep in mind that it's your business, and you're likely taking most of the risk. Don't haphazardly offer equity partnerships in the business too soon. Reserve those options for those you know well and who have proven themselves to be valuable contributors to your company.

SECTION THREE

Insanely Valuable
Need-to-Knows

CHAPTER EIGHT

REGULATORY AND LEGAL PLANNING: AVOIDING THE PITFALLS THAT COULD SET YOU BACK

"If opportunity doesn't knock, build a door."

—*Milton Berle*

I thought it was too good to be true. I was almost dreading the idea of checking to see how he was doing. I really wanted to believe that this could work. But if I wanted to go ahead with my plans, I really didn't have a choice. So I opened the browser and started my search.

I was Googling the name of the ER physician who had originally planted the seed in my brain to open a ketamine therapy clinic. Yes, this is the same physician I had a conversation with years earlier when he was opening his clinic. Now I was gathering information with the idea of opening my own.

To be honest, I was skeptical that he was having success with such a niche practice. Not to mention that the treatment wasn't covered by insurance, which in my mind, greatly limited its potential. I could almost taste the bitter disappointment in my mouth as I typed his name into the search bar when gathering information about how his practice was doing.

To my surprise, not only had this physician moved his clinic to a bigger space but he was also getting ready to open his third clinic! I couldn't believe that he was doing so well. My anticipatory disappointment transmuted into exuberant enthusiasm. I was practically dancing when I told my wife about it.

However, my excitement started to fade as I began to research what went into opening a clinic. The opportunity was definitely there, but there was so much to learn. The more research I did, the more I wanted to open the clinic, but I wasn't able to find any training programs or consultants that specialized in helping providers open niche self-pay private practices.

There were so many rules and regulations. I struggled to piece everything together and was dumbfounded when I realized that there was absolutely no central source for any of the information I needed.

I did a lot of Googling and spent hours and hours digging through websites to find answers. I looked at the websites for my state's Department of Health, the Board of Nursing, the Board of Medicine, the Board of Pharmacy, and the Drug Enforcement Administration to see what was required for private clinic licensure.

I called the Board of Pharmacy multiple times and read all the articles I could find. The guidelines from prominent nursing organization websites indicated that I lived in a state where CRNAs could practice independently. I was working in a hospital without the direct supervision of a physician, so that seemed to make sense. All these things led me to believe that I could start my own clinic and independently treat the patients in my practice.

When we finally opened our doors, everything was off to a great start. We had patients calling to set appointments left and right. We were growing week after week. (Cue scary music.) But that complaint filed by the nearby competitor was really causing me a lot of stress.

Inside, I was panicking. Was my clinic going to be shut down? Would I lose my license? What if there was disciplinary action against my license and I had to explain that in every job interview I applied to in the future? Will this cause me to get kicked out of the Navy Reserves? Would I have to pay back the student loans the Navy Reserves helped me pay?

My mind was racing with every possible worst-case scenario it could think of. I had just started celebrating that I had opened a clinic and now I might have to close everything down.

This competitor had looked at my website and didn't see any notation of a collaborating physician on my clinic's webpage, and this was why he reported me to the Board of Nursing. Even though multiple nursing organizations stated on their websites that New Mexico was an independent practice state, I found out much later that there was indeed language in the New Mexico

Nurse Practice Act (NPA) that said a certified registered nurse anesthetist *"shall collaborate"* with a licensed physician. It turns out that many nursing organizations like to over-exaggerate the level of independence APRNs have in some states by blurring their definitions of what independent practice is. I was in a heap of trouble.

The state's Nurse Practice Act reigned supreme and the New Mexico NPA said I needed physician collaboration. The reason this had never come up in the hospital is because we always discussed the cases with the surgeon ahead of time and they were always standing a few feet away from us during surgery. Physician collaboration happened as part of the day-to-day job.

Unfortunately for me, the Board of Nursing's attorney was out for blood. He was clearly trying to make an example of me. During the several months surrounding this ordeal, I was unbelievably stressed out, wondering if I was going to lose my clinic—or even worse, my license.

Through this experience, I learned that attorneys who work for licensing Boards function in a way that is similar to criminal prosecutors. They get bragging rights, awards, and promotions based on how many "criminals" they take down. These state licensing Boards and their Board members are typically political appointees. Nothing says "we are doing a great job" to the governor who appointed them more than keeping a tally of all the healthcare professionals they have disciplined for infractions or alleged infractions.

If you ever find yourself in a similar situation, never communicate with these attorneys without first consulting your own healthcare attorney who specializes in license defense. The state licensing Boards and their staff are not your friends, colleagues, or anything of the sort. They are not there to help you. In most states, they provide little to no guidance or assistance because they are in the business of "protecting the public." They do not exist to serve the legal needs or questions of licensed clinicians, period.

This fiasco ended up costing thousands in attorney's fees and many sleepless nights. Thanks to a lucky break that resulted from a desperate letter I wrote to the Board members pleading for leniency, I was offered an official "Warning Letter." I received notice of this letter the same day that I was about to accept a "plea deal" from the Board's attorney. Had I accepted the deal, I would have had my license both formally disciplined and put on probation.

Thankfully, with the help of an experienced attorney who specializes in exactly this kind of law, we gathered proof that authoritative nursing resources stated misleading information on their websites and falsely indicated that New Mexico was an independent-practice state.

As a result of immediately owning up to my error, offering a valid explanation, and preemptively taking CE training courses to show them I was actively pursuing a better understanding of scope of practice, I got off with that official warning. I promise you this stroke of luck only happened by the grace of God.

It turned out that the solution for my practice was pretty straightforward. I either needed a physician to collaborate with so that I could continue to practice and prescribe ketamine for pain, or I could hire a nurse practitioner. So hiring a nurse practitioner is what I did, and I was able to keep my clinic open and growing.

The lessons? Always hire an attorney, and know your state's laws and regulations. This is one of the areas you do not want to brush off. Find a highly skilled and experienced attorney licensed in your state to ensure you have structured everything related to your practice in a way that is compliant and mitigates risks to the greatest reasonable extent.

Federal, State, and Local Regulations

Regulations are broken down into federal, state, and local. Federal regulations apply to everyone. State regulations apply to those in the state. And local regulations apply to a specific area of the state. Your attorney will help you make sure that you're not missing anything.

Federal Regulations. There are some important caveats in play with federal regulations. Some of the rules that apply to practices that accept insurance are different from the rules that apply to self-pay clinics. Get familiar with federal regulations to know what is allowed.

State Regulations. Make sure that you are allowed to own a practice in your state with your license type. In most cases, anybody who has to take an exam to become a licensed medical professional qualifies and can own a practice. Some states make it compulsory for a physician to own the practice but there is always a workaround.

Local Regulations. Zoning is the main item to check for when it comes to county or city regulations. These rules indicate where commercial activity can take place. Make sure you are in an area that is zoned for a medical practice. Check with your local zoning office for more information. If you're in the boundaries of a specific city, your city might have its own set of zoning, apart from the county. The property appraiser's office can usually tell you which zoning regulations apply specifically to your business.

Licensing, Regulations, and Legal Planning

Licensing, regulations, and legal planning are some of the most intimidating topics to think about when starting a clinic. But fear not, these things are simpler than you might imagine.

Any information in this book related to licensing, rules, and regulations is accurate as of the writing of this book. But keep in mind that things change frequently. If you take the time to learn and understand everything you can and then meet with an experienced attorney to review the latest information available for your state, you will have nothing to stress about.

Business licenses are required by all states and are easy to get. Just go online and type in your state and register with a local tax collector. You pay a fee and give them the basics: your business name, address, and business type. You may also need to register this license with the Department of State.

In most states, you have to post your business license somewhere that will be easy for the public to view. It is required that you renew the license every year so the municipality knows who is doing business in their jurisdiction.

Most states allow a clinic to be operated under the license of the provider who owns the practice as long as they are licensed in that state and practicing in the clinic. This may mean that there is an exemption for a state *medical clinic, medical facility, or healthcare facility license*. I used three descriptors there because states that require those types of licenses tend to use different nomenclature.

There are a lot of rules and regulations that people don't even know exist and it's never really a problem and can easily go unnoticed—at least initially. To know the rules, you need to know the rule makers. There are different regulatory bodies that ensure every practice or business follows the regulations imposed by these bodies.

Occupational Safety and Health Act (OSHA)

The Occupational Safety and Health Act (OSHA) is an organization established by federal law that applies to all physical places of business in the US. It exists to make sure work environments are safe for those who are there. You know those big posters you see in any business that outline health and safety regulations? That's OSHA. It sets standards and provides training, outreach, and educational assistance.

Employers must follow relevant OSHA safety and health standards and must be able to find and correct any safety or health hazards. There is information that you must provide to your employees and contractors. Inform them about chemical hazards through training, proper labeling, alarms, and color-coded systems. Specific to the medical field, OSHA has requirements for blood-borne pathogens among other healthcare-related topics. There's a medical and dental office's guide to compliance on their website that has all the details.

An important thing to be aware of is the MSDS, which stands for Material Safety Data Sheets. To be compliant, you will get a binder and list all of the hazardous chemicals, disinfectants, and cleaners in your office. Inside the binder, you also have instructions about what somebody should do if they ingest any of these things or are otherwise exposed to toxic chemicals. And yes, this includes common home or office cleaning supplies. That binder should be in a place where your employees can find it in an emergency.

Medical practices also have to provide medical or personal protective equipment (PPE). This includes equipment to protect the skin or eyes, prevent respiratory exposure, and so on. You'll have to provide an eyewash station or eye irrigation kit with a complete first-aid kit.

If you invite an OSHA inspector out, they'll tell you exactly what you need. The inspectors that arrive when you are proactively requesting an inspection aren't there to be punitive. Their goal is to help you be compliant, so don't be afraid to invite them in.

Centers for Disease Control (CDC)

The Centers for Disease Control (CDC) puts out recommendations for infection control and guidelines for outpatient settings. You can get a PDF of a guide specifically for outpatient practices.

It's not a list of regulations, per se, but their disease control guidelines are considered a standard of care. The guide also includes a checklist. If you're a licensed healthcare professional with experience, you're going to be familiar with most of it, but it is a good idea to review it anyway.

The Clinical Laboratory Improvement Amendments (CLIA)

All facilities in the United States that perform laboratory testing on human specimens for health assessment or the diagnosis, prevention, or treatment of disease are regulated under the Clinical Laboratory Improvement Amendments of 1988 (CLIA).

Basically, if you're running any test on any sample that is collected from a human patient, you need to have a CLIA *certificate* or a *certificate of waiver*. Let's say you're processing a lab that qualifies for a CLIA waiver, such as a urine dipstick pregnancy test, or a finger-stick blood glucose test; the clinic would be waived and therefore only needs a *certificate of waiver*.

A comprehensive list of lab tests that qualify for a CLIA *certificate of waiver* can be found on the FDA.gov website. Just to be clear, even though you are offering these waived lab tests, you do have to obtain a *certificate of waiver* and keep it up-to-date. You have to renew it every two years, and they will charge you a small fee to do so.

Drug Enforcement Administration (DEA)

The Drug Enforcement Administration (DEA) requires that healthcare providers dispensing or ordering controlled substances must obtain a DEA license. According to the DEA website, an individual practitioner with a DEA license who plans to dispense or order controlled substances does not need to obtain a separate license for their clinic as long as they place their clinic address on their license. Most practitioners that have been practicing will already have a DEA license.

Physicians will have a Practitioner License, most other prescribers will have what they call a Mid Level Practitioner License. If you don't already have one and plan to prescribe controlled substances, apply for it and enter your clinic address on the application. If you're not a provider, then you will need to apply for a hospital/clinic DEA license.

If you have to apply for your DEA license, apply early. It can take several weeks to obtain your first one. You don't want this to hold up your clinic opening. Your state may require you to have a state-level controlled substance license. Get it first, or the DEA will deny your application. Check with your state Board of Pharmacy to see if you need a controlled substance license for your state.

The DEA license number assigned to the holder of the DEA license will be used to order controlled substances for the practice. Whoever's license is being utilized to order for the clinic is ultimately going to be responsible for ensuring that the clinic is properly handling, documenting, and disposing of any controlled substances. Sometimes this alone is reason enough for a clinic to obtain its own hospital/clinic DEA license.

Licensing with Boards of Healthcare Professionals

These are the agencies you want to investigate while looking through your state licenses and your state license requirements. The titles of these organizations vary slightly in terms of the wording or name but they are going to be the first places to look when you're trying to figure out if you need a special clinic permit or a clinic inspection.

Make yourself aware of the different rules that exist for the boards in your state. When making inquiries and calling the different departments and organizations, ask them if there's anything else you should know when starting a private practice.

Remember, these Boards do not exist to help you or to provide legal advice. Some may not even answer basic questions. If someone does answer your questions DO NOT misinterpret any help or advice they provide as a substitute for legal advice. You may be talking to a secretary who is simply trying to be helpful but may have limited knowledge of the rules or regulations.

Any information obtained should be fact-checked and you should confirm it is accurate. Some states have very strict rules when it comes to "outpatient infusion clinics." Typically, when you hear about seemingly over-complicated rules or regulations related to an infusion clinic, they're talking about freestanding and chemotherapy-type outpatient infusion clinics.

Get to know the terminology and the exact legal definitions that your state uses. This is another area your attorney can help you with.

Department of Health

Departments of Health differ by state. In general, these departments create rules, regulations, licenses and policies related to the general health of the public and the treatment of health conditions.

When you talk to this board about your plans to start a private practice, be sure to mention if you are a licensed healthcare professional. The rules and regulations can be very different for somebody who wants to open a medical practice when they have a professional healthcare license versus when they don't. If you don't make this clear to the Department of Health (or its equivalent) they might classify your clinic incorrectly. When it comes to rules and regulations, the devil is in the details.

When I called the Board, they assumed I didn't have any healthcare training or a healthcare license. They immediately told me I need an assortment of facility licenses, facility certifications, permits, and more. The application for a facility license had a tremendous amount of requirements, including building blueprints, minimum square footage, and even hiring a pharmacist.

It turned out I didn't actually need any of it because I was a licensed healthcare provider. If I hadn't caught onto the differences, I would have put a lot of time and money into getting a bevy of expensive licenses that I didn't need.

Board of Nursing

If you're an APRN or RN, go to your state's Board of Nursing website to look up the Nurse Practice Act (NPA) and make sure you will be practicing within your scope. The NPA will tell you what kind of agreement with a physician, if any, you should have—for instance, a collaboration agreement or supervising agreement.

Board of Medicine

If you're a physician, check with your Board of Medicine to make sure there aren't any special requirements that need to be met to start a practice. If you are a physician and you think you're going to hire a nurse of any type, you will also want to go to the Board of Nursing website and read the NPA.

You want to understand if you must be physically present in the clinic when other providers are providing care. You also want to ensure that you are allowed to oversee the type of care being provided. For example, an obstetrician/gynecologist physician may not be able to provide routine non-STD-related care for male patients. If scope of practice rules like this exist in your state, you want to know about them before starting your practice and caring for patients.

Board of Pharmacy

Some states require you to have a pharmacist as a consultant. There are states that require pharmacists to do an inspection or to review your pharmaceutical handbook to make sure that you have appropriate policies to order, store, and handle your medications.

Keep in mind that private clinics often have fewer restrictions and fewer requirements than healthcare facilities, so you'll want to make sure that you're describing how your practice ownership is structured to avoid being classified wrongly. This is yet another place where your attorney comes in handy.

Other Licensing Boards

It is common for Doctors of Chiropractic Medicine (DC), Doctors of Oriental Medicine (DOM), and other licensed health and wellness professionals to start private clinics. Since they are not classified as *providers*, their scope of practice is limited. They are not able to do things such as prescribe medications or provide other services that MDs and DOs can provide.

Again, it is important for these professionals to understand what treatments and care they are allowed to personally provide and what treatments and care need to be performed by a licensed provider.

For example, in most states, DCs and DOMs are not authorized to personally prescribe or provide IV therapy, so they hire a provider such as an APRN, PA, or physician who can prescribe and administer these treatments. Each type of healthcare professional must be intimately familiar with exactly what they are allowed to do.

CHAPTER NINE

INCORPORATION: THE "WHY" AND THE "HOW"

"For every minute spent organizing, one hour is earned."

—*Ben Franklin*

Once you have hired your accountant and attorney, start getting organized. Organization is vital to the success of your practice. So stop, buy a three-ring binder, three-ring hole puncher, some paper, and some divider tabs. Yes, I am going old school.

Make a legal tab, an accounting tab, and an incorporation tab. Keep the binder with you whenever and wherever you do any official business. If you go to the bank, take the binder with you because they're going to ask you for your incorporation and IRS documents.

You will also need the documents in the future for tax returns and a variety of different business activities. You do not want to lose them. If you go to the bank and open up a bank account, they may want the actual physical papers. For certain transactions, you will even be required to present the originals. You want to keep a backup in electronic format, but you should always have the hard copy of everything, and you should keep originals in your corporate binder at all times.

It's time to incorporate. Incorporation is crucial because it provides tax advantages and liability protection. If your business ever gets involved in a dispute or lawsuit, you will have a "corporate veil of protection." This is a mysterious-sounding phrase to describe a level of protection that guards your private assets and anything that you hold personally.

Being incorporated helps shield you and your personal assets from future business debt, liabilities, errors, or omissions resulting from mistakes the business, employees, or contractors of the business could make or be accused of making.

You'll hear about things like C corporations, S corporations, Limited Liability Corporations (LLCs), Professional Corporations (PCs), Professional Limited Liability Corporations (PLLCs), and others. Each corporation has different tax, accounting, legal, and documentation implications. Here's a rundown of the different types of corporations.

Corporation

For tax purposes, there are two types of corporations: C corps and S corps. It's unlikely that a clinic owner would want a C corporation status because these are subject to double taxation. The corporate profits/dividends are taxed as well as the income that's paid out to the owners. In many cases, small business owners who established a corporation elect to be treated as an S corp. All corporations that are established are initially C corporations. To get tax treatment as an S corp, you will have to file form 2553 with the IRS. This is where accountants and attorneys become vital to helping you save money in taxes and penalties. You want to have your accountant and your attorney in place before you start to set these entities up.

An S corp is known as a "pass-through" entity. This means that corporate profits and losses are actually passed right on to the shareholders, and they go straight to the personal shareholders' tax returns. In an S corp, the taxes are only paid once, and the owners of the company pay the tax at the individual level on their personal tax returns. Corporations are administratively more complex than LLCs or sole proprietorships.

An attorney can help you create all these legal and administrative documents. Into your binder they go. Just so you know, you're supposed to have annual meetings that are documented, aka take minutes (put those in your binder, too) to help get the protection of that corporate veil. Simply set a recurring evening in your calendar to hold an annual meeting. If you fail to meet the administrative requirements, then you set yourself up for personal liability.

Limited Liability Corporation (LLC)

In this structure, business income and losses are also passed on to corporate shareholders' personal tax returns on a schedule. An LLC can elect to be taxed as an S corp. It is a common entity choice for private practice owners if a different entity choice isn't required by their state.

Some states require a professional corporation, which is a PC or PLLC. Not all states recognize these professional corporations, but some require that certain licensed healthcare professionals operate as such. These states have their own regulations related to this. In some cases, all shareholders are expected to have a certain license type.

These professional corporations can be the choice for professionals who work in medicine, accounting, law, or engineering. One benefit is that the additional owners are typically protected from malpractice claims against any partners of the corporation.

Do It Right

A word of advice: once you file the incorporation documents, beware of scammers. They send mailings that look like they're coming from the government. They'll talk about things like mandatory certificates of incorporation, or they will sell you wildly overpriced labor law posters and all sorts of related scams.

If in doubt, call your state agency before you buy something. The scammers use seals that look similar to state seals and make it look like they're coming from a state agency. Prepare for it.

If you're paying for legal fees for incorporation, you will find that an attorney will likely charge you anywhere from $400-$700 just for the initial consultation. Some might charge you as much as $3,000 or even more to have a corporation fully set up for you. That's about how much I paid when establishing a corporation.

In my own case, the attorney created a binder with every document that I needed and took care of absolutely everything. She even gave me checklists to make sure she explained all the state requirements. For me, that was worth it. I had peace of mind knowing that everything was being set up properly and that I knew exactly what was required for administrative compliance.

Understanding the Scope of Practice

There's a simple three-step process to understand the scope of practice regulations if you're a licensed healthcare professional. If you're a physician, pay attention, because you need to know this when you hire an advanced practice nurse or any other type of healthcare professional.

If you hire an APRN and they're practicing outside their scope, you as the business owner can potentially be held liable. While these steps will help you to navigate and understand your local laws, still consult an attorney before opening up your clinic.

Step 1: Let's say you are a licensed nurse. Google your state plus your exact license type plus the words "practice act" or "scope of practice." Look for the link that goes to your state's licensing board website.

If you are a nurse, this would be the Board of Nursing website. Download the Nurse Practice Act, and read the entire thing word-for-word. The document will tell you exactly what you can do with your license type in your state.

If you're an APRN living in a state where you don't need physician oversight, you can run a clinic entirely on your own with just your license. If you're having trouble deciphering your NPA, don't worry. You are not alone. They can be extremely vague. Write down the sections you find regarding the scope of practice related to your license type. You'll need it in step two.

Step 2: Determine if you need any physician oversight. If you do, is it physician supervision? Or is it just physician collaboration? If it is collaboration, does there have to be a written collaboration agreement or can it be verbal collaboration? Or are you an independent provider who can provide care without physician involvement?

The laws can be complicated, and they can sometimes have additional regulations located within other areas of state law. The only way to truly protect yourself is by paying an attorney who is familiar with medical case law, scope of practice law, and healthcare law to guide you. The worst thing you can do is follow some article on the internet or take a coworker's advice as fact.

Most states that require supervision for APRNs do not require the physician to actually be present at the clinic. In these states, the physician has to have a license in the state where you are practicing and be available by phone or email for consultations.

Step 3: If you are not authorized as an independent provider, find yourself one. Just to refresh, in case you forgot, a provider is a physician, a physician assistant, or an APRN. Each has scope of practice rules that they must adhere to. Physicians are independent providers in every state; they don't have to do anything in this step. If you're not a provider at all, say maybe you're an RN, find a provider to evaluate the patients, develop the treatment plan and write the orders.

If you live in a Corporate Practice of Medicine (CPOM) state and you need to hire a provider, often a physician is required. You may have to give away ownership of the clinical side of the business. The exact nuances and details of that setup are outside the scope of this book. I gave one short example in Myth #8, but you'll need a good attorney to walk you through that process. You'll just have to understand if your state is a CPOM state and how that impacts your license type.

Possible Pitfalls

There are a lot of regulations when it comes to pain management, including scope of practice regulations. The opioid epidemic made many states add strict regulations on pain management clinics. In some states, only physicians are allowed to provide pain management services.

Advertising the treatment of pain can automatically classify you under state laws, as a pain management clinic, which means you would have to abide by all the laws of a pain management practice. So be careful, do not advertise that you're treating pain until you talk to an attorney, or review these laws. In Florida, the Nurse Practice Act also states that a nurse of any type cannot advertise that a controlled substance is being administered or prescribed. So be very careful with the additional rules and regulations that encompass pain management and controlled substances.

Marketing Compliance

Marketing compliance is put in place to ensure that when you sell or market products and services, you are marketing in a way that's not misleading or downright dishonest. Simply by doing what's right and ethical, most healthcare professionals won't have anything to worry about here. Making exaggerated claims that are non-factual, lacking evidence, misleading, or flat-out lies are the things that can get you or your clinic in serious trouble.

Marketing compliance comes in the form of Federal Trade Commission (FTC) and FDA rules and regulations. We aren't going to get into the weeds on this topic, but you should be aware of some common pitfalls.

You can learn more about FTC regulations by visiting ftc.gov or ftc.gov/legal-library. Here you can find all sorts of legal cases and proceedings that have been documented as examples of what *not* to do. It's not a bad idea to do a little research on the site to see the types of cases that are made against practices that were offering services similar to your clinic.

Most compliance rules are reasonable. For example, with regard to FDA approval, the Agency for Healthcare Research and Quality (AHRQ) states that: "Off-label prescribing is when a provider prescribes a drug that the FDA has approved to treat a condition different from what the FDA initially approved it for. This practice of off-label prescribing is both legal and common. In fact, one in five prescriptions written today are for off-label use."[4]

When providing a non-FDA-approved treatment or prescribing medication for non-FDA approved indications, the fact that it is

---

[4] Carolyn M. Clancy, "Off-Label Drugs: What You Need to Know," Agency for Healthcare Research and Quality, (U.S. Department of Health and Human Services, September 2015), https://www.ahrq.gov/patients-consumers/patient-involvement/off-label-drug-usage.html.

non-FDA approved simply needs to be presented conspicuously on a clinic's website and other marketing materials, in addition to having the provider disclose this while getting the patient's consent. It should also be written on the consent that the patient will sign.

When your marketing describes the results a patient may get, that is considered "making a claim." So if a clinician or clinic owner claims that a treatment is going to produce a specific result or outcome in their marketing, it is important to cite a study or studies that validate that claim.

One of the biggest mistakes that a clinic that offers vitamins or supplements can do is to claim a vitamin or supplement can *treat* or *cure* a disease on their marketing material or product labels. The FDA and FTC aggressively pursue those who make false or unsubstantiated claims related to vitamins, supplements, products, or treatments.

CHAPTER TEN

INSURANCE: PROTECTING YOURSELF FROM THE UNKNOWN

"The only way to deal with risk is to understand it, quantify it, and manage it."

—*Mark Twain*

Proper insurance will help to reduce your financial risk exposure and protect you from unpredictable events. As a wise business owner, you'll want to insure your business, your entire staff, yourself, and your family.

Practice owners commonly purchase various types of insurance, including malpractice, business, unemployment, workers comp, disability, and umbrella insurances. They're technically separate, but sometimes insurance companies will offer a bundle the same way your cable, phone, and internet can be bundled.

Picking the Right Insurance Company

Not all insurance companies are created equal. Search the web and the Better Business Bureau (BBB) for reviews. It's also important to look at the rating of the insurance company to know how strong they are. The largest rating companies include A.M. Best, Fitch, Kroll Bond Rating Agency (KBRA), Moody's, and Standard & Poor's. Each has its own rating scale. To use the ratings from more than one independent agency, you need to understand that each agency's rating code is different from the others. For example, an A+ from A.M. Best is the next-to-top rating of its 15 categories, but an A+ from Fitch, Kroll or S&P is their 5th-highest rating.

The highest ratings demonstrate that they have the capital in reserves to pay out claims when they come due.

An A+ or a better rating demonstrates that they have the capital in reserves to pay out claims when they come due. If you were to use a company that isn't financially strong, it could go out of business, and you would be exposed to extra financial risk.

Choose a solid company that's been around for a long time and has a good reputation for taking care of its customers. The last thing you want is to get cheap coverage from a fly-by-night company that loads their policies with exclusions so they don't have to pay claims.

When you're looking at insurance, note that most professional organizations will likely provide some sort of referral to a specific carrier. There isn't anything inherently wrong with that, but you should know that organizations commonly receive a commission or some other type of financial remuneration for recommending a company or product. In other words, it is likely a biased recommendation. The same can be true for insurance brokers; some may only recommend products that pay the highest commission.

Word to the wise: insurance can be a bit of a double-edged sword. If there is ever an allegation against your business, "in-a-wreck-get-a-check" attorneys (these are the guys on the billboards all over your city) will specifically attempt to gain information about your insurance and policy limits as quickly as possible. They do this to determine if a target is valuable enough to pursue. They are after one thing: money.

More insurance coverage equals a potentially bigger payout for them. Most of these attorneys/law firms keep at least 30–35% of everything they "win" for their clients. That means a $5 million dollar settlement with the insurance company would earn them a cool $1.5 million+.

They will often file lawsuits just to attempt to get a settlement—especially on smaller value lawsuits—because it can cost the insurance company several hundred thousand dollars to defend against an allegation. If there isn't much to gain (aka your insurance coverage isn't robust), there is less chance that a suit will be brought against you.

If your personal income is well above average, let's say $400k+ per year, and/or your personal net worth is over $2 million, you had better get extra coverage because you can *personally* become a target. If and when you get to this level of personal wealth, I would highly recommend consulting with a personal asset protection attorney.

It is important you know which insurances are required and which ones may be optional to avoid purchasing unnecessary coverage. The top four required insurances are listed below:

Medical Malpractice Insurance

Medical malpractice insurance is mandatory for licensed healthcare professionals. The rates will vary greatly depending on the type of license the provider holds, the amount of coverage needed, and the state in which one is practicing. Some states have tort laws favorable for clinicians and other states have tort laws that create more payout risks for the malpractice carriers.

It is advisable to get coverage that includes legal fees for any sort of Board investigation or any complaints against your professional license. When it comes to coverage amounts, most states set the minimum coverage that a clinician is required to have as part of their malpractice policy.

States like New Mexico have state-managed patient compensation funds. If you buy into the fund, there are also statutory limits on the dollar amount that a provider or medical professional can be held liable for when it comes to malpractice claims. Look into state-managed funds and other programs your state may have in place to help encourage medical professionals to practice there.

Options like these could save you money and help reduce your risk exposure, but it is important to understand how they work.

Some may appear to be great values, but when you start to read the details, you may find that they aren't really that great.

Some malpractice carriers include pages full of limitations or exclusions, so it's important that you go through your documents to make sure that you are going to be covered for the services you plan to offer.

One thing to keep in mind is that you want to add your corporate entity to your malpractice policy. If a lawsuit were ever to be filed, or any claim ever to be made against you or your practice, a plaintiff will almost always include your practice (aka your business entity) in a lawsuit.

Medical malpractice attorneys are like vultures circling the sky, looking for what could become a feeding frenzy. I can guarantee you that they will be looking for as many people and entities to place their alleged blame on. In other words, they are seeking more bank accounts, assets, and insurance policies to prey upon.

Don't set yourself up for the possibility of personal liability. Always insure everything related to the business, including the business itself. A lot of times there isn't even an additional cost to add the business.

Group Malpractice Policy

As your business grows, look into getting a group malpractice policy. That way, you can make sure that everybody in your practice has malpractice insurance, including you, the owner, and the business entity. It's also less costly to add various staff to one policy than to have them purchase their own individual malpractice insurance.

It is often easiest to obtain this type of policy when all the clinicians are of the same specialty. If you plan to provide coverage for staff that has a variety of license types and specialty types, you will likely need to find an insurance broker that specializes in this type of coverage.

No matter which type of coverage you have, be sure you save the documentation of all the insurance coverages for you and your business. Sometimes lawsuits and insurance claims can get made years after an event, and if there is no saved documentation of who your insurance provider was and who was covered, you could be setting yourself up for risk.

Speaking of a claim being made years later, you may want to consider only purchasing occurrence policies. With this type of policy, the claim can be reported anytime after an alleged event and the insurance company will still provide coverage.

Contrast that with a claims-made policy where a claim must be filed when the policy is in effect in order for the insurance to provide any coverage. If the holder of a claims-made policy purchased a tail-coverage policy, this would provide coverage for any claims that might result from a complaint made in the future, after the policy expired. In other words, if you purchase a claims-made policy, *always* purchase tail coverage before the policy expires or lapses. Failure to do so creates major liability issues.

General Business Insurance

Business insurance coverage protects businesses from losses due to events that may occur during the normal course of business. There are several types of insurance for businesses including coverage for property damage, legal liability, and employee-related incidents.

As a business owner, you will evaluate your insurance needs based on potential risks, which can change depending on a variety of variables like location, method of service delivery, services offered, and others.

At the minimum, property insurance and general liability insurance are must-haves. Most major insurance carriers carry specific policies that bundle multiple business coverages together. Most bundled plans like these are going to cover you in at least these two major categories.

Property

If you are leasing an office space, you will want property insurance that is going to protect your equipment, signage, inventory, and furniture in the event of an unexpected accident or tragedy such as a fire, storm, vandalism, or theft.

There's a good chance that your landlord will require that you have a certain amount of property insurance. If you are leasing, ask your landlord what their business property insurance requirements are and make sure you meet them. If you own the building, then you will have additional coverage for the building itself along with other contents of the building.

General Liability Insurance

General liability insurance helps cover the cost of injury and property damage claims against a business. It can help pay for medical care, repairing or replacing damaged property, and legal fees for covered claims. It covers things that happen within your practice that are unrelated to the medical care that is being provided.

Let's say somebody spills a cup of water on the clinic floor, but your staff doesn't see it because they're in the other room. Then somebody walks through the front door, slips on the water, and breaks their hip. They'll probably expect the clinic to pay for their medical bills. If the clinic refuses, they might sue. They will claim the injury was a result of negligence because the business didn't clean up the spill fast enough.

An attorney would argue that the business should have known that the floor was wet and someone in the business should have marked the hazard or dried it up quickly to prevent a fall. Accidents and injuries (real or alleged) like these are what general liability insurance helps protect your business from.

Workers' Compensation Insurance

Every state requires you to have workers' compensation insurance if you have any W-2 employees. Some states allow a business to buy into a state-sponsored workers' compensation insurance fund, while in other states, you will need to contact a worker's compensation licensed agent to purchase it.

In some states, if you're the only person working in your clinic as you start up, and you're the sole owner of that practice, you can make yourself exempt from having to purchase the compensation for yourself. But as soon as you get a W-2 employee, you have to have it. Your accountant will usually have pretty good recommendations in this area. Your payroll company will have recommendations as well.

Almost all states require businesses to put up a poster describing the company's workers' compensation insurance. Many payroll companies have one that they'll give to you for free. Free or not, you will have to post this information in the break room, an area that meets the required criteria, or an area where employees tend to congregate.

"Great-to-Have" Policies Include:

Cyber Liability Insurance

Cyber liability insurance protects your business from the cost of cyber threats or breaches involving computer systems and data. Cyber liability insurance helps protect your business from vital data breaches that can happen through your company computer or network. The data could be the patient's, the business's financial data, or anything else that can be stored electronically.

Data breaches can potentially result in hefty fines and legal fees. If you decide you want this type of coverage, it is critically important to ensure you purchase a policy that doesn't have exclusions related to HIPAA violations because some policies will attempt to carve out coverage for HIPAA-related breaches.

Commercial Umbrella

Commercial umbrella insurance provides an extra layer of liability protection. It complements your other liability coverages by kicking in when your other liability coverage limits have been reached.

It is important to note that this coverage is not at all related to the professional services that you provide and the malpractice coverage you carry. It serves as another level of security above and beyond things like your commercial car, business liability, and property insurance, among others.

These types of policies will specify the exact baseline coverage your business must maintain. It is critical that the business always carries those baseline levels of coverage because the umbrella policy only takes effect once those baseline policies have been maxed.

Reducing Risks and Being Prepared for Emergencies

For a business, you will want to invest in training your employees for emergencies. We have created a Policies and Procedures manual that has different policies for a variety of scenarios. This 540+ page P&P template manual is included in all our training programs. To learn more about our training programs and all the forms and templates we include, head here:

jasonduprat.com/book

A good emergency policy concisely highlights important information, for instance, where people meet if there's a fire. Proper actions to take in the event of an emergency should be spelled out, and each employee should be trained on them.

I recommend putting together your own manual, storing it in an easily accessible place, and letting everyone know where it is.

Everyone should have the opportunity to read through it and have easy access to it at all times.

There are medical emergencies you want to be prepared for too. Problems could arise from things like adverse side effects or complications related to a treatment that you offer. Be sure to have a clear protocol for the treatment as well as the appropriate medications and people to treat that emergency. Otherwise, it could look like you knew a treatment you were performing could potentially be very harmful to a patient, but you didn't have the proper precautions in place.

What happens if someone were to give too much blood pressure medication intravenously and their blood pressure drops dangerously low? What are they going to do to fix that? They could cause serious injury or death by administering a treatment incorrectly. What if the patient has an adverse reaction to a medication? You must have everything in place to quickly and efficiently attend to every possible emergency.

Everything at a Glance

There are basic rules and regulations that surround starting and owning a practice. Knowing them saves you time and money but most importantly, it saves you from getting in the type of trouble that could cripple your business before it even begins (not to mention potential harm to a patient).

Some rules apply generally, while others depend on the state you're in. Again, I would advise you to hire professionals (attorneys, consultants, etc.) who know what they are doing and can point you in the right direction. Got it? Now it's time to get started.

SECTION FOUR

Getting Started: Excited? You Should Be!

CHAPTER ELEVEN

SELECTING THE PERFECT OFFICE SPACE ON A BUDGET

"The most important aspect of a successful business is its location."

—*Sam Walton*

I couldn't help her. We went back and forth for a while as I tried to understand her situation. The RN I was speaking to had partnered up with a physician to start a medical clinic. She had huge goals and aspirations, but what she made up for in enthusiasm, she lacked in experience.

She wanted her clients to get the best of the best, which is no bad thing, but one of the first things she did was go out and sign a lease for a beautiful 6,000-square-foot clinic space in Manhattan. Brand new, brand name equipment, lavish furniture, ritzy decor ... She spent an ungodly amount of money to open—well over a quarter million dollars. Her clinic was growing, but she spent so much upfront she could hardly afford to run the practice anymore.

She maxed out several business credit cards without realizing she'd be personally liable for the debt. She was so new to business, her plan was, "If this doesn't work out, the business will just file for bankruptcy, and that'll wipe out all of its debt." When push came to shove, she called me to see if I could help her turn the clinic around.

She started too big, and she didn't have a proper understanding of business financing or how bankruptcy works. Starting a business with large amounts of debt and using bankruptcy as the exit plan may seem like a bad idea to you and me, but what it came down to is that she didn't know what she didn't know.

It's important to get proper education and coaching to minimize the pool of unknowns when opening your business. Start-up is the most crucial time in your company's life. With so much riding on the line, you want to account for as many of the variables as you can.

Besides reading books like this, I'd strongly recommend surrounding yourself with other clinic owners who can help you and answer any questions you have along the way. You may not know what you don't know, but they probably do.

All of my clinic start-up training programs include access not only to our instructors, who are also clinic owners, but also to our private student communities. These are filled with hundreds of other healthcare professionals and clinic owners that can serve as sounding boards and informal advisors to guide you on your journey.

I also host a mastermind exclusively for clinic owners who are aspiring to build multi-million-dollar practices. This mastermind aims to foster collective growth of all its participants. There is a culture of collaboration and idea sharing unlike anything else out there. This is a program for those who desire to be the best of the best. Access is limited to only one clinic per area. You can learn more about this exclusive mastermind here:

jasonduprat.com/book

Regardless of whether or not you join one of my programs, remember to always pass it forward; if you receive help or advice, give help and advice to others. Choose to become the mentor for the next aspiring clinic owner who is looking for guidance. And, bonus for you: by teaching others, you'll become a *true* expert.

The Location

Choosing an office location is one of the most important decisions you will make when starting a clinic. It can potentially make or break your practice. Once you sign a lease, you are usually committed to that location for a minimum of one year and often for as many as three to five years.

We discussed honing in on a location in a previous chapter. There we focused on how to find the most viable city or town to get started. Now, let's discuss what goes into actually narrowing down the exact location.

Once you have done your analyses and narrowed down your choice of city or town, you need to determine which specific neighborhood will produce the greatest likelihood of success. There are several factors to consider when choosing the most suitable place for your clinic, such as:

- Location relevant to competitors
- Ease of access to highways
- Security and safety
- Property costs
- Parking

It's probably a good idea to position yourself in a different area of the city from competitors. We aren't opening a Starbucks— you don't want to open up two blocks down the street from a rival clinic.

Look for locations near a major highway, airport, train, or bus station. I know it sounds like we're planning a getaway for a heist, but the salient point is that if your clientele could be coming from far away, the easier it is to access your clinic, the better.

While talking about access to the clinic, we can't ignore the parking situation. Unless you are downtown in a major metropolis like New York City, you need to have plenty of parking. Having limited on-street parking is a deterrent to business in most areas, especially if some of your patients are dependent on wheelchairs for mobility. They will need handicapped parking right up near the building. It will be a big problem if your patients can't find parking and then when they do, they can't easily get out of their vehicles. They might come once, but they likely won't come back.

Your location should be in a clean and safe part of town. Even if you find a beautiful building and cheap rent in an area with higher-than-average criminal activity, you are setting yourself up for more headaches down the road.

You might have expensive equipment, or you may even be storing controlled substances. Don't make your clinic a target by placing it in a less-than-desirable part of town. Keep security and safety in the back of your mind when choosing your exact location.

Sometimes, neighborhoods can change quite drastically as soon as the sun goes down. Drive by prospective locations in the evening to gauge the environment. Look at the lighting and behavior of people outside after dark.

Do you see people standing on the street? How about large numbers of cars stopping in the street to "talk" to the guy standing on the corner all day? Be on the lookout for worrisome behavior. If in doubt, look deeper or move on.

A good way to gauge if a building is the right one for you is to do some reconnaissance. Ask the other tenants about their experience. It doesn't take long, and you might find some valuable information. Some questions you might ask are:

- What are your thoughts about the building? Do you like it?
- How long has your business been renting here?
- Are the landlords friendly?
- Do they fix the problems that come up? How fast do they fix them?

- What's the noise level outside and inside?
- Can you hear loud noises through the wall?
- Is there any fine print in the lease that you didn't know of until afterward?

The intelligence you gather from doing this could save you from unforeseen problems. Most people are friendly and enjoy helping others, especially if you might be a future neighbor. Don't be afraid to get out there and ask around.

Sometimes gifting a dozen bagels can go a long way to not only making friends in the building but also getting them to tell you everything you could possibly want to know about the landlord and management company.

The Exterior

So, you've found a location that may work. Stand in front of it. This is what your patients will see when they arrive at your clinic. Look at the overall condition of the building. Is the paint peeling? Are there large cracks in the building? What is the condition of the parking lot? What is the landscaping like? The first impression really matters.

People will judge whether or not they want to visit your practice based on what they see from the parking lot. If there are any substantial problems affecting the outward appearance of the building, either negotiate with the landlord to take care of them or move on to the next potential location.

Exterior signage is another important consideration. You want your patients to be able to find you. Is there already a monument sign in front of the building that you will add your clinic's name to, or do you need to build your own signage? Who will pay for it?

Unless you are planning for a high volume of walk-in patients, it's unnecessary to purchase costly oversized exterior signage. If your patients will be making appointments, then there is a good chance that they are going to be using Google maps to find your office. As long as it is reasonably easy to find and has visible signage, patients should find you without difficulty.

Another important consideration for the outside of the building is lighting. If you plan on working into the evening when it's dark, make sure the area surrounding the building and the parking lot are very well-lit.

Ask the landlord what time the outdoor lights turn on. Good exterior lighting goes a long way in providing a safe space. Not to mention peace of mind when you are walking to your vehicle alone in the evening.

The Interior

Security isn't just an exterior concern. It's important to make sure you keep your employees, your patients, your business, and yourself as safe as possible. Ask if the building has security cameras, automatic locking doors, and other features to increase safety and security.

One thing that may help in this endeavor is to put your office on the second floor, or above, of a medical office building. It makes it much more challenging for somebody with criminal intent to force entry into your office.

Remember, since anything above ground level is less accessible, an elevator is a must. When I was looking for my space, there was a beautiful place that I fell in love with. I didn't see an elevator though and when I asked about it, it turned out the building didn't even have one. It was an automatic no-go. If I hadn't asked, they probably would not have mentioned it to me.

There are more than just safety and accessibility concerns to be aware of when you're looking at the interior of the office or building. Here are some other major things to be thinking about when inspecting the space your business may call "home":

- The aesthetics of the interior of the building matter a great deal. Take a look at the walls. Are they well painted, with no scuffs, holes, or chipped paint? Are the light covers free from dust and dead bugs? How well does the inside of the building appear to be maintained?

- Are there restrooms in your office? If yes, where? If not, how far are they from your office? You will need a handwashing sink. Is there one in the office you're looking at? Can one be installed?

- You also have to consider storage. When you inspect the interior location, make sure enough storage is available. Where will you stock your medical and office supplies?

Size Matters

When it comes to the size of the office space you lease, consider your income goals, goals for your practice, the size of your market, the population, your startup budget, and your risk tolerance.

When I started, a low-budget, lean startup was the only option. I knew the practice could always be scaled up afterward if we saw that it was successful. That way, the risk would be minimal if things didn't work out. I've said it before, but it's worth reiterating. In most cases—especially if you're bootstrapping and new to business—starting small and lean is going to be the way to go.

But, if you're a Warren Buffet or know someone who is, and they are willing to inject a large amount of capital along with years of business experience, you may want to consider a different strategy. Hitting the market quickly with a large clinic with the capacity to expand and build out multiple locations within a short period of time could be an option for those experienced in business.

Reid Hoffman, co-founder of LinkedIn, calls this strategy blitz scaling. Without very large investors and a highly experienced team, getting too big too fast would be detrimental to most. If you don't have the funds, team, and experience, it is usually best to stick to the start-small-and-grow strategy.

CHAPTER TWELVE

CRACK THE CODE: UNDERSTANDING COMMERCIAL LEASES

"The art of negotiation is not about getting what you want; it's about getting what you need."

—*Chris Voss*

There are a couple of different ways a lease is usually offered for a commercial space. The first one is a standard tenant landlord lease. Obviously, this is an agreement where a tenant is leasing directly from a landlord.

The second one is a sublease. That's not a hard one to figure out, either. Someone else leases directly from the landlord and then they turn around and sublease you a portion of their already-leased space.

If you're going to sublease, just make sure that the person or business subleasing to you has an agreement with the landlord that contractually allows them to do so. Otherwise, you risk being evicted by the landlord once they find out (and they always find out).

Types of Commercial Leases

Okay … now here's when we get to the juicy stuff … Just kidding! The main thing about commercial real estate leases is that they are organized around two different rent calculation methods: net lease and gross lease. Then there's what you get when those two leases have a couple few drinks and get to know each other better. A bouncing baby modified gross lease, which combines features of the two.

Gross Lease

The rent is all-inclusive in a gross lease. The landlord takes almost all of the expenses associated with the property, including the taxes, insurance, and maintenance out of the rent that the tenants pay.

It may even include janitorial services and utilities, all bundled into this lump sum, tenant-friendly rent payment option. When negotiating, definitely ask if the janitorial services are included, and if so, what that entails. There are different levels of janitorial service—it could cover common areas only or it could include the interior of your office space. It is common for utilities to be included with a gross lease, but excessive utility consumption can be charged back to the tenant.

This is one of the best leases for a startup because you can easily predict your monthly expenses and won't have to pay extra costs associated with other types of leases. Plus, the landlord will assume responsibility for all the extraneous expenses related to the building. As you may imagine, this type of lease is not easy to find and is typically only offered with Class B or C real estate or in slow economic times.

Net Lease

Initially, a net lease will look more attractive as it has a lower base rental rate. The landlord charges a lower rent for the space, but there are many extra expenses you will be responsible for.

These are usually costs associated with the operation and maintenance of the building, but they could even include real estate taxes, property insurance, common area maintenance, janitorial services, property management fees, sewer fees, water, trash collection, landscaping, parking lot maintenance, sprinkler maintenance, and any other expense the landlord may wish to spread out among all their tenants. So be one hundred percent sure you know exactly what you will be paying for and how high those costs could potentially climb.

Be aware that there are several different kinds of net leases. These include single net, double net, and triple net. As you move from single net to triple net the tenant becomes increasingly responsible for expenses related to the building. If you're looking at signing a net lease, just make sure you know what you're getting into.

Modified Gross Lease

The modified gross is more tenant-friendly than a net lease and is a compromise for the convenience of both parties involved. It will be your base rent plus a standard flat fee to help cover some of the expenses related to the property. Make sure you know what the flat fee covers and what it doesn't—and know how much those things cost.

Making Your Lease Offer

When we were first looking for a space, we were looking for the ideal, perfect location that was already set up exactly the way we wanted it to be. What we actually found in our budget was just an open room that had a sink and a closet. It needed work. A lot of work.

At the very least, we had to rip out the carpet, paint, and put up a divider wall. Luckily, we used a broker who specialized in helping people find commercial real estate. She helped walk me through the transaction and even suggested requesting that the landlord provide funds for tenant improvements to offset the cost of the work we needed to put in.

The landlord agreed to cover half the cost of painting, new flooring, and the installation of the divider wall. The landlord ended up paying for around $3,000-worth of improvements. Not a bad ROI on simply asking, right? We never would have known to negotiate if the real estate broker hadn't suggested we make the request.

Never accept any initial terms they present to you without asking for something more favorable to you and your business—something with more concessions. Negotiations are customary in commercial leasing. Some landlords inflate their rents and fees in anticipation of being asked to come down in price during their negotiations.

Present yourself and your business as an ideal candidate for tenancy, one worthy of concessions. Be professional about your counter offer and clear on the rate you'll pay, the length of the lease, and the renewal options.

Make sure you have the renewal options in writing, which provides you the ability to renew that space before your original lease is up. Also, include any improvements you want to complete.

When searching for a commercial location, enlisting the help of a commercial real estate broker or agent is very advantageous. This is true even if you are renting and not purchasing a location. The agent or broker will be compensated by the seller or lessor for assisting with the rental of a commercial property. There is typically no cost to you as the renter of a commercial property.

Brokers and agents know the area and they can often see listings before they get published on the major commercial real estate websites. It will reduce the time and energy you will spend searching. Also, in many cases, the broker can help you learn what the prevailing market rates are for various property classes and locations.

CHAPTER THIRTEEN

SUPPLIES AND EQUIPMENT: CRUCIAL DETAILS YOU NEED TO KNOW

"The only thing constant in business is change, and the only thing you can control is your own expenses."

—Barbara Corcoran

You have two options when purchasing equipment: new or used. Be prepared to pay top dollar for new equipment, especially if it is brand-name. If you search online, you can find used, refurbished, or generic equipment for just a fraction of the price. Online stores like eBay and Amazon are great resources to check for inexpensive equipment.

Exercise good judgment here. Purchasing invasive equipment like lasers or surgical devices for example is best done through licensed vendors in the United States. Blood pressure machines, and monitors, along with other simple, non-invasive equipment can be purchased safely online as long as it is inspected for proper functionality and safety by a licensed biomedical equipment service company or technician. There are also several auction websites and websites that specialize in refurbished equipment that can provide you with a great deal of savings.

As a small practice owner, I typically recommend buying generic, used, or refurbished whenever possible because the cost savings are tremendous. As a lean startup, I was looking to save expenses wherever it was safe and reasonable to do so. However, for some clinicians having additional peace of mind makes it worth paying more; and some may prefer the warranties and service contracts that may be included when purchasing new equipment. If that's your preference and you have the funds, by all means, go right ahead.

We purchased brand new, generic cardiac monitors off of eBay that cost us around $550 each. We ordered three at once and were able to negotiate the price. You could pay $2,000 to $6,000 for a Philips or a GE cardiac monitor that has similar functionality. Even if the cheaper models break and you have to replace them every few years, you still come out ahead.

If you're purchasing refurbished equipment through a third party, some manufacturers consider the warranties null and void if they aren't repurchased through licensed resellers.

Large healthcare institutions usually have their own biomedical department to maintain the equipment. Smaller institutions tend to outsource their biomedical needs, but they'll always run tests to make sure it's calibrated and gives accurate readings. Before you put any used equipment into service, have a biomedical company inspect it, certify it and put their sticker on it. God forbid, you buy something used off the internet, don't get it inspected, and you get the wrong reading on a device, which influences patient care, or worse, sets your whole practice on fire. Failing to properly test and inspect used equipment can expose you and your practice to increased liability.

One option we haven't addressed yet is renting equipment. You can rent a lot of the more expensive equipment that you may need. The great part about renting is that you are often not responsible for maintenance and repairs. Now, there are exceptions, be sure to read your equipment lease contract so that you understand exactly which party pays for various repairs and maintenance. This is critical when it comes to renting costly machines like lasers. Make sure to add likely repair and maintenance expenses to your operating budget.

Keep your patients' mobility and accessibility in mind when choosing your equipment and furniture. For instance, we had to purchase chairs patients could sit in while getting infusions. These were all comfortable recliners. To ensure our larger patients felt safe and comfortable, we made sure to have at least one recliner that was extra-sturdy and large. This made the experience better for our bariatric patients and patients who were over 6-feet tall.

Many clinic owners choose to purchase consumer-grade furniture because medical-grade equipment that is aesthetically pleasing is very hard to come by. If you go the route of consumer-grade equipment, be sure to analyze them for fall hazards.

Don't get recliners that rock, swivel, or lay too far backward. They are difficult to get out of, and if they have a rocking or swivel function that can't be locked, it will create an unstable support when your patients use them to push themselves up and out of the chair. This is especially true of obese and older clientele. We don't want people falling and breaking any bones.

Distributors

There are many different sources where you can get your medical supplies. There are national distributions, as well as regional, and local distributors. Our training programs include a comprehensive list of preferred medical and pharmaceutical distributors and we have secured several discounts that are not available to the general public. To learn more about our training programs visit:

jasonduprat.com/book

To start, you will want to create a list of distributors that are available in your area. If you are working at a healthcare facility, go ask the managers or department heads where they order supplies from. You may also want to ask other clinic owners in your area.

Occasionally you can find a little gem of a local or regional distributor that may offer better service or better delivery options. Sometimes these smaller vendors will have items that are out of stock or back ordered at the larger distributors.

You can also check the stock room of your hospital, clinic, outpatient surgery center, or wherever you may be, and write down manufacturer names that are printed on the supplies. You can also add to your list by searching online for medical supply distributors in your area.

In every industry, some distributors are better than others. Do your research, read reviews, and ask other practitioners before making your first purchase to ensure you're getting a good deal and not being taken advantage of.

My clinic used Medline, and we found them to be a great source. They're a big manufacturer, but they're also a distributor. Because they make and sell their own products they tend to have some really good prices. However, they do not have pharmaceuticals. Some medical suppliers will have pharmaceuticals, and others will not. Same thing with controlled substances.

Quick note: Amazon sells medical supplies, although they don't sell pharmaceuticals as of the writing of this book. They are reportedly entering the pharmaceutical space soon.

There are a handful of things you want to consider when you're choosing which vendors you're going to order from. Certainly, price is a huge deal. Other things to take into consideration are shipping costs, quality of service, how fast they deliver, and availability of their products.

One thing you might not have thought about is how honest they are. This is a question you should intentionally seek the answer to. A vendor's level of integrity is very important. I've run across some dishonest and unethical medical distributors out there.

I highly recommend that you open up multiple accounts with several different vendors to do some price checking. This also helps with backorders. It's surprising how many vendors are continuously out of products. Opening multiple accounts helps to ensure you can get the supplies you need when you need them.

Shipping

Shipping costs can vary dramatically from distributor to distributor. Some of these companies charge absolutely outrageous shipping charges. The only way to know what they charge is to go through an entire order. I would suggest putting together an order and simulating a checkout. Go all the way to the last step to find out how much they're going to charge you, including shipping.

If you're ordering over a certain number of dollars, a lot of companies will give you a break on the shipping. They might even ship your order for free. So consider consolidating your orders, and place one or maybe two a month. This takes a little bit of extra planning. This can be done by setting a Periodic Automatic Replacement (PAR) level.

Most established, well-run practices set a PAR level for their medical supplies and pharmaceutical inventory. Your PAR level is the minimum amount of inventory needed to meet the demand from your customers while providing a cushion in case of unexpected demand. Of course, that level will be substantially higher for things you go through quickly than for something you may use a few times per year.

Establishing a PAR level will also help you systemize your business. Unless you have electronic inventory management, have your entire supply checklist printed out or in a spreadsheet, including the PAR level. That way anybody, including the receptionist, can place orders.

If you're supposed to have three cases of 20 gauge IVs on the shelf and they only see one, they know to order two. This takes you out of the equation. Anything that gets you closer to the goal of a business that can run without you is a big win.

Using this system will also help you save money over the long term because you'll be able to order some items in bulk and you'll save on shipping. Above all, setting a PAR level means that you won't be looking for an IV start kit when you need it, only to find you're all out.

Ordering Controlled Substances

Many medical supplies distributors also sell pharmaceuticals. Some pharmaceutical companies sell controlled substances and some do not. You will have to do some research to find out. If a vendor is either making or distributing controlled substances, they have to have a DEA license. There are standards to which they have to adhere and they are inspected and shut down pretty quickly if they're not doing things by the book.

Be prepared to go through a thorough credentialing process when you place your first order of controlled substances. You will have to show your professional licenses, your DEA license, and your state-controlled substance license (if your state requires one), and they may even ask you for your business licenses and a description of your clinic activities.

I actually had a bit of trouble with this. When we started ordering for the practice, the address on my DEA license listed the hospital where I was working as a CRNA. When I placed the order, the location I was ordering for (my clinic) didn't match the address on my DEA license. It caused a pretty big delay. I actually had to update and order a new DEA license and it took several weeks to get it. Lesson learned. Make sure all your paperwork is in order and you have crossed the *t*'s and dotted the *i*'s.

The controlled substance distributor asked for a written statement describing the controlled substance that I would be ordering, what they would be administered for, along with an estimate of the number of orders I would be placing and the quantity of product those orders would be for.

It may seem extreme, but there are regulations that state that the distributor has to *know their customer.* To know a customer, they have to know the customer's ordering habits. So if you make a drastic change in your ordering habits, call to let them know ahead of time, or they may report you to the DEA for atypical ordering practices.

Going back to our ketamine clinic example, let's say you normally order two cases of ketamine a month but you hear there might be a shortage coming. If you place an online order for eight cases without sending an updated form first, there's a good chance the DEA will show up at your door and ask you what the extra ketamine is for.

It's best to order directly from a sales representative. If you actually call to talk to the sales rep, they will often be able to give you discounts over the phone that you can't get by ordering online. Once you go through the rigamarole of placing your first order, your subsequent orders are usually very simple and very routine.

CHAPTER FOURTEEN

HUMAN RESOURCES: YOUR BOOM OR DOOM

*"I would rather hire a person with enthusiasm and teach
them the skills, than hire someone with the skills and try
to instill enthusiasm in them."*

—*Zig Ziglar*

As a brand new clinic owner, you are likely doing mostly
everything. But all of that is about to change. Okay, yes, you
also have to don the Director of Human Resources hat now, but
you won't be wearing all these hats soon. The first few employees you hire will probably be an additional provider, your front
office receptionist, virtual assistant, or maybe some back office or
clinical staff. Some clinics start with one versatile person who can
help cover multiple roles.

Your goal should be to transition out of the *jack-of-all-trades*
role as soon as it is financially possible. You own the business, it
shouldn't own you. It should be able to run without you. That's
where real *freedom* comes in.

As you become a savvy entrepreneur, you will quickly see that your time is too valuable to wear all the hats in the clinic. For some, that will happen within a couple of days or weeks. For others, that process may be drawn out.

If you are a provider, your highest value is not in micromanaging or taking on every role in the business. Your biggest ROI is delivered when you see patients, perform procedures, write orders, and oversee infusions. And eventually, you may choose to hire someone else to take over your *provider* role, as well.

Hiring—Work "ON" Your Practice, Not "IN" Your Practice

Remember the complaint that our competitor lodged against us? Because of it, we had to find a nurse practitioner as quickly as possible or shut our entire practice down.

After interviewing only three candidates for the job, we hired someone hastily. Her references and background check were fine, but she was a little rough around the edges. Long story short, she just didn't show up one day. We found out later that she had stolen a prescription pad that had my clinic's name on it and was writing controlled substance prescriptions for a family member. This was discovered when a pharmacist from across the state called to notify me about her suspicious prescribing.

In hindsight, I can say we had missed some small clues. She didn't speak very professionally. She was a heavy smoker, and when she would chat, she would frequently talk about her fondness for drinking alcohol. Those were red flags that I overlooked. Be cautious, and don't ever ignore red flags—even if you are in a bind.

Hiring great staff can be a challenge. The biggest and best piece of advice I can give you is not to wait until you're overwhelmed to fill the required position. If you do, it will cause you to sacrifice or compromise your standards. The worst thing you can do is bring in somebody who is subpar. It will be detrimental to your business. Give yourself enough time for proper screening to ensure you bring the right type of staff with the right values into your practice.

Before you begin hiring, it's important to have job descriptions in place. The potential employees need to know the position they're interviewing for before the interview begins. Otherwise, there will be a lot of room for miscommunication and ambiguity. State everything the job entails and what you're looking for very clearly, in writing.

Job descriptions also help protect you as the employer. If an employee is not performing the duties written in their job description, it helps you have a more solid legal foundation to terminate an employee who's not performing well.

Another important point to make here is when you are making an offer to a potential W-2 employee, you, as the employer, are responsible for half of the 15.3% FICA (Federal Income Contribution Act) tax the government will collect on this person's wage. That means on top of the salary you will pay the employee, you will be paying the government 7.65%. Don't forget to factor that in, plus there are other employment costs like worker's compensation and unemployment insurance. If your offer is $100 an hour for a W2 employee, you will more likely pay $115-$120 per hour out of pocket.

FICA tax works differently for independent contractors. The contractor pays the entire 15.3% of FICA tax themselves. Make sure that in their 1099 contract, it is very clear that the contractor pays their own FICA tax in your employment or contract agreements. You don't want to end up in a situation where the tax goes unpaid by the contractor. This is yet another reason why an attorney is so important.

Be sure to ask your accountant if you are required to pay yourself as a W-2 employee of your company. How much to pay yourself is something you should also discuss with your accountant.

Nursing Staff

Whether you are hiring a nurse or any other licensed healthcare professional, verify their experience, get references, verify their license, and all their certifications and credentials. You also want to ensure that everybody being hired for a specific role has those specific duties within their scope of practice in your state.

For example, Botox comes up a lot in clinics, and in some states, nurses can't administer Botox. It's very odd, but there are a few states where the person administering the Botox has to be a provider like a nurse practitioner or a doctor. There are rules like these for many procedures. Similar rules exist for who can perform procedures with laser equipment. Make sure you know them.

Receptionist

A receptionist is one of your most important hires. This employee will be the public's first interaction with your practice. If they greet your patients, answer your phone, and schedule appointments in a very nice, pleasant way, it goes a long way toward getting referrals.

Ideally, you will find an intelligent, happy-go-lucky person who is constantly smiling and has impeccable customer service skills. I have had the unpleasant experience of facing a rude, grumpy, and condescending receptionist at many medical offices. I am sure it is relatable to almost everyone. So, if you want your clinic to do very well, you cannot accept anything but the absolute best for this position.

Some clinics may have patient populations with particular needs. Our practices had mental health patients, as do many other ketamine practices. These patients often have an added level of vulnerability and anxiety. With these kinds of patients, the person at the front desk is especially key.

Find someone who can be calming and reassuring. If your patients do not feel genuinely warm and welcomed as they approach and interact with your clinic, they will not return, and will possibly leave negative feedback on review sites.

Your receptionist must be able to represent you and your practice well, and they must ensure that your patients receive outstanding customer service because anything less should not be tolerated. It may require you to pay above average for your area, but it's well worth it.

Office Manager

You will probably not have the revenue to hire a top-notch, full-time office manager/practice manager until your clinic is a little bit more established. The best office managers are pretty darn expensive. They are going to expect full-time hours and benefits packages.

You may want to start by looking at part-time office managers or maybe healthcare professionals with some management experience. You may even be able to offload some typical office manager duties to a high-quality receptionist. A great receptionist might be able to take on some of the administrative responsibilities, and they might be able to run reports and help decrease the administrative load.

It's not a bad idea for you to take on this role yourself in the beginning, especially if you are not seeing a whole lot of patients. Managing your own practice means you will have substantial savings on labor expenses, plus you will gain a lot of valuable operational insight. You'll be familiar with all the systems (or lack thereof), patient communications, and any scheduling breakdowns.

In addition, at least initially, you will be at the forefront of your operations. As a result, you will be able to work out the kinks in your processes to make sure that your clinic is operating as smoothly as possible. Decide which roles you want to outsource, and which positions you want to keep in-house or want to take on yourself. The key is to leave yourself a substantial amount of time and energy to work on your practice.

Provider

You may also need to find a provider or maybe you need a supervising physician for your practice. The best place to start is your network. If you work in a hospital or clinic already, there's likely someone you know well that could be a potential provider or supervising physician. In many cases, it's as easy as asking them.

Start networking through Facebook groups or LinkedIn if you can't find anyone in your personal network. You can also post the position on an online job site like Indeed or LinkedIn. As I mentioned earlier in the book, there are also some companies that specialize in providing supervising physicians for those who need or want them.

Policies and Procedures
Employment Agreements
Contracts for physicians, providers, and even other employees should be prepared and reviewed by an attorney with experience in employment and healthcare law. These contracts can potentially be costly, especially provider-level agreements.

The good thing is that employment contracts can be reused for years to come. There are a lot of statutes and regulations that they're ruled by. It's important that they're all taken into consideration or your clinic can end up in employment disputes. Certain violations can even result in fines.

If possible, you want those provider-level agreements to include non-competition and non-solicitation clauses. It is not uncommon for the providers to seek employment at a type of practice they eventually intend to start on their own.

We had a provider apply who wanted to start a ketamine practice, and she thought she would use us to get paid on-the-job training, then quit to start her own practice. For that reason, you have to get those good non-competes in there and protect your-self from every angle. Be aware that non-compete clauses are not legal or enforceable in all states.

You also want to ensure your contracts protect any providers from stealing your patients, intellectual property, physical property, or otherwise causing your clinic harm. List out the types of offenses that are grounds for immediate termination. Your attorney will know your state laws and what would be included.

Have a Progressive Disciplinary Action Policy in Place

Make sure you have a progressive disciplinary action plan in place. Many states have a lot of requirements to help reduce the risk of harassment or discrimination against employees. It is paramount to document poor performance through a pro-gressive disciplinary action policy. This should document how you're coaching, counseling, and working toward getting your employees to perform the duties according to what is outlined in their job description.

If you get frustrated with an employee and terminate them on the spot—especially if you don't have a documented track record of coaching and progressive discipline prior to their termina-tion—you set yourself up for discrimination allegations.

On the other hand, if the track record and job description reflect that you have taken all the appropriate steps to encourage and train your employee to do the right thing before firing them, you will have solid ground to stand on. When you terminate someone, having all those documents helps to protect you from a potential future lawsuit.

There are some cases where you can terminate an employee immediately, but you always have to consult with an attorney. For instance, if they show up to the job drunk or lose their license to practice, you do not need to document a progressive disciplinary action plan with them. If you ever run into a situation like this, or one where you aren't sure, rather than terminating them on the spot, send them home first. Then immediately consult an attorney.

Employee Handbook

A lot of the items we have discussed will be part of your employee handbook. Among other things, this handbook should contain privacy policies, HR-related policies and procedures, and job descriptions. It's true that creating policies and procedures is a pretty time-consuming task, but it's a good idea to have them in place before the clinic opens, especially if you won't be in the practice 100% of the time it's operational.

There are companies that provide a variety of HR services and many payroll companies also offer them as add-on services. There are companies that will help you write your employee handbook for an additional fee. They typically have templates that you can customize yourself, as a less expensive option. Check to see what your payroll company offers and start customizing your handbooks based on their recommendations, especially if they can help you with state-specific regulations. Our training programs also include HR-related policies and procedures along with employee handbook templates that can be customized.

Payroll

As the owner of the company, you are ultimately responsible for everything in your business. This includes ensuring that all of your payroll taxes and payroll-related expenses are paid.

You may be aware that when it comes to taxes, there is more than just the FICA tax that we mentioned earlier. Some states have their own tax, some counties have their own tax, and some cities have their own tax.

If you miss your tax payments, you have to pay late fees, penalties, and usually interest on top of that. It can get really expensive really fast if you miss any deadlines. Way more expensive than just paying a payroll company and an accountant for advice. This is why I strongly recommend getting a good accountant or CPA and using a specialized payroll service. It's essential that the person taking care of these things knows what they're doing.

On top of taxes, there are two major payroll-related insurances you have to maintain: unemployment and workers' compensation insurance. Payroll companies can set it all up for you, pay the premiums, and file any reports required by the state.

Some full-service companies are Paychex, ADP, and OnPay. They all have multiple packages that include a variety of different products and services. If you're already using QuickBooks accounting software, they also have a payroll service, and it's incorporated right into their software for accounting. There are many other companies, big and small. Do your research to find the right one for you.

You Still Have to Work

Even though you have a payroll company, it doesn't mean you get to completely ignore it. There's still some work to do. You have to submit your employees' hours. Typically, payroll companies give you a certain deadline before which you have to submit your hours for each employee or each contractor.

Remember, the buck stops with you. You still have to understand what goes into payroll because you have to ensure it is being done properly. To do this, you have to obtain the reports from the payroll company.

If they're making tax deposits on your behalf, you have to know how to go into their software system and get printouts of those payments and reports. Review them monthly or quarterly to make sure that the payments are being made correctly.

You will also have to determine your payroll cycle. Are your employees going to get paid weekly, bi-weekly, or monthly? Your payroll company will help you determine your payroll scheduling.

Payroll companies do negotiate their prices. I was able to negotiate Paychex down twice on their fees. You might be able to negotiate upfront or you might try negotiating down the road. Now that there's a lot more competition in this payroll space, these companies are more willing to work with you on price to keep you as a customer.

Retention Incentives

Offering a profit-share is one way to retain key employees, but there are other ways you could achieve the same goal. You could offer larger 401(k) company contributions, more attractive competitive packages, larger salaries, or more vacation time.

The best thing you can do is to create a fantastic work environment where people love coming to work. Showing employees that they are valued isn't just a decent human thing to do, it is also a good business practice and will reduce the chances that they will want to leave.

SECTION FIVE

Next Steps: Roll Up Your Sleeves and Get Ready to Crush It

STREAMLINING: HOW TO STAND OUT AND MAKE YOUR COMPETITORS IRRELEVANT

"Streamlining is not about doing less, it's about doing more, faster and with fewer resources."

—David Allen

My first degree was in hotel and resort management. During and after graduating with this degree, I worked in restaurants and hotels. I enjoyed hospitality and learned a lot from the business model. So, when I thought about opening my clinic and the experience I wanted my patients to have, it was a non-negotiable to bring a customer-centered service model into my practice. As we streamlined our processes, we always kept the patients in mind.

When you streamline something, you are optimizing various parts of your business to eliminate errors or sub-optimal patient or employee experiences. It helps you avoid and reduce the possible problems, errors, or hiccups that can occur. It's usually an iterative process where you're constantly making small tweaks and improvements to correct for little errors or issues that appear in operational processes along the way.

Streamlining aims to create an efficient model that makes every part of the practice run more smoothly. It has the happy dual advantage of reducing your operating costs while increasing customer and employee satisfaction. And, as you know, these two groups of people are key to the success and longevity of any business. You want to keep them happy.

When it comes to patients, it's always about delivering high quality care and an outstanding experience. Everyone involved wants their care to be as quick, easy, and pleasant as possible. When you have exceptional service, you stand out. The word will get out very quickly and you'll easily attract an influx of patients.

Customer-centric streamlining gave me a competitive edge when I first opened. Patients started flocking to my clinic … and running away from my competitor. From what those patients told me, the provider who ran the other clinic did not really care about the patient experience. The patients weren't satisfied with the service he provided, but they didn't have any other choice. He was the only game in town. When I opened up, patients left his practice in droves. The most effective business strategy is to simply strive to be the absolute best at what you do.

I have seen other clinic owners focusing their time on thinking about how to attack or take down the competition by filing complaints, leaving fake negative reviews, or other unbecoming tactics. This type of behavior takes time away from making mean-ingful improvements in one's own clinic and if done dishonestly or with malice, it can even be grounds for a lawsuit. Focusing on your competition is purely a distraction. If you focus your efforts on being great instead of on how to "take down" the competi-tion, you're setting yourself up for the best probability of success.

Let's face it, self-pay patients can choose to go anywhere they want. There's a big difference between successfully operating a cash-based practice versus an insurance-based practice. Since these patients are paying out of pocket, they expect, even demand, a much higher quality of service, and rightfully so.

If you have been to a Ritz Carlton or other luxury hotel or res-taurant, you know exactly what I am talking about. My first-ever Ritz Carlton dining experience is a perfect example of focusing on the customer. I was speaking at a multi-day conference and went to their hotel restaurant for lunch. The server was very friendly and great at building rapport, the service was excellent, the food tasted great and was prepared very quickly, and my bev-erage was never more than half empty.

I had a good experience the first time, so the next day I decided to return. Not only did the server immediately remember my name but he also recalled my exact order from the previous day. He even asked me if I would like the grilled cheese with tomato soup and unsweetened iced tea again *or* if I would like the menu to try something new.

I was stunned that he remembered—he had many custom-ers the day before. He had greeted me instantly upon entering the restaurant, so he didn't have time to go and look at notes or orders from the previous day. It was impressive and it made me feel *special*.

You should strive to be the Ritz Carlton of medical practices. You should strive to make every single patient feel *special*. To do this, you need to map out the entire customer journey—from the first time they hear about your clinic, to the first time they receive care, all the way to their return visit. Every single detail of every interaction with your practice should be mapped out.

You need to put a great deal of time into thinking about how you can create a "WOW" experience at every step of their journey. If you do this well, you will be able to make your competition irrelevant.

Systems

Almost every process or department in a business can be streamlined through software tools and applications. You could streamline your accounting process by subscribing to software like QuickBooks and linking it directly to your business bank account. This could save you the stress and time of manually categorizing transactions and it can reduce bookkeeping errors.

Something amazing happens when you focus on creating smooth efficient processes. You gain a tremendous amount of headspace. It prevents you from expending mental energy by putting out the day-to-day fires that are ignited when good systems and processes are not in place. When you free up your mental bandwidth, your patient interactions can proceed unimpeded by nagging thoughts about administrative to-do's. You can leverage that freed-up headspace to work on the business and plan for growth instead of being trapped in fixing the little day-to-day problems.

By creating systems, you can find shortcuts, invent ways for things to go more smoothly, and maximize efficiency while also standardizing quality. Basically, any step of a process you do regularly that has a set of tasks that don't change can be worked into a system. The more basic the system, the better. Never underestimate the value of a good checklist. It's beautiful. It's simple.

Let's say you're onboarding a new hire. There's paperwork that needs to be done, materials that need to be read, and training they need to complete. You can create a checklist that you use every time you're onboarding a new hire to make sure you don't miss anything.

You could use checklists for things such as:

- Appointment setting
- Patient check-in
- Patient check-out
- Patient follow-up
- Chart reviews
- Payroll
- Collecting payments
- Report generation

What other things do you think would benefit from having a standardized process created for them? When you have a system, you don't have to think about what has to happen to get x, y,

z done. You just whip out your handy-dandy checklist and—
voila!—you can get it done in a cinch. Or, better yet, give someone else the checklist and rest assured that they are doing the job
exactly the way you would want it done.

Using Policies and Procedures to Streamline Your Clinic's Operations

Policies and procedures are the business owner's way of documenting how things should be. If you think about policies as the
"why" you do something, then procedures would be the "how."

If you're a solo practitioner and have no employees, you need
policies, but not as critically as those running a full-scale business. When your business involves a team of people delivering
a product or service on your behalf, policies become critical to
ensure that patient care and clinic operations are happening
consistently every time. The goal is to ensure that everybody is
following documented policies and procedures so, at the end of
the day, the desired outcomes are achieved.

Take, for example, how great restaurants prepare their food. The
best restaurants have a recipe card—the procedure—that details
the ingredients and preparation steps that every chef has to follow. Everything is measured down to the gram and each step is
to be executed precisely.

The restaurant may also have policies that describe exactly which
vendors the restaurant orders all of its food from and may even
specify the exact brand of mozzarella to order. That way, no matter which chef is working, your lasagna will always taste exactly the

same. The service is always exceptional because all the chefs, the wait staff, and the management follow the same procedures every time.

Put procedures in place to make sure your patients and employees know what steps to take. It will massively increase the odds of getting a consistent outcome. When you start listing out the policies and procedures you should have at your clinic, the list can get really long.

For human resources, you'll want to map out how vacation is accrued, how and when time off should be requested, and how sick days are accrued.

For urgent situations, you'll need emergency policies and procedures. For example, where does staff meet in the event they need to evacuate? And who is responsible for ensuring the patients also get out?

Clinical policies and procedures will determine which patients qualify for an IV insertion. There should be a step-by-step procedure that describes how to safely and correctly insert an IV. Tools like these are critical for risk mitigation.

You'll need policies for other medical or nursing procedures. There could be a policy detailing when a central line can be accessed in your clinic and the qualifications required to provide that service. A central line access procedure would again detail the exact steps the clinical staff need to complete to sterilely access a patient's central line.

Another example of a policy for an aesthetics clinic might be one that states "Botox must never be administered to patients that

are allergic to botulinum toxin products or to any of the components in the formulation. It should never be administered in the
presence of infection at the proposed injection site(s), or to any
patient with a neuromuscular disease."

Policies like these are designed to ensure that only appropriate
patients are getting treated. They serve as one of many layers of risk
reduction that a clinic owner uses to reduce the possibility of errors.

When it comes to clinical procedures, the best policies and procedures should include medical and nursing references. This
should be a citation to a textbook, journal article, or published
guideline that was used to detail the particular steps outlined in
the procedure checklist.

As part of our business accelerator training programs, we have created a clinic Policy & Procedure manual template. It is designed
to accelerate the process of creating what is needed from scratch.
We advise reviewing and customizing it for your practice and the
services offered at your practice.

To learn more about all the amazing resources contained within
our training programs, visit:

jasonduprat.com/book

Using Policies and Procedures to Streamline Your Customer Experience

Being a customer-centered clinic is about paying attention to
what it's like to be a patient. If you're empathetic and put yourself
in the patient's shoes, customer needs are hard to miss.

Little mistakes can be easy to make in the beginning. Sometimes, a clinic won't think to have a policy about notifying the provider that a patient is waiting in a given room, so the patient could be sitting there for a very long time, wondering why they were waiting so long. New clinic owners tend to make small mistakes like these because they have a lot going on and haven't carefully planned outpatient flow.

When there aren't proper systems in place, problems in customer service and even patient care can arise. If too many of these happen or they aren't promptly corrected, you may end up in a situation where you have received several bad online reviews and are forced to dig yourself out of a negative PR hole.

At any point where you have a delay in care or a hiccup in patient flow or worse—an upset patient on your hands—you have to pause and do a root cause analysis. Ask yourself these questions:

- "What happened in the lead-up to this issue?"
- "What caused the problem?"
- "What can we do better next time?"

In the provider notification example, you could then come up with a system like putting the patient's chart on the door facing vertically to indicate to the provider that the patient hasn't been seen. When the provider sees the patient and comes out, he could flip the chart sideways.

Some clinics have colored exam room door flags and if a certain color is flipped out, it means there's a patient needing to see the provider. If high-tech is more your thing, then there are a variety of clinic software tools that can be implemented and used.

You can incorporate a variety of tools to make service delivery and the patient experience as smooth as possible. The key to ensuring that any system or process is consistently followed is to create the policies and procedures for them as well as provide proper training for your staff.

Another way to improve the customer experience using policies is to eliminate any chances of overbooking. It is a common problem clinics tend to run into, and it does not help anybody.

Once you have a practice, you should have a reasonable estimate of the number of patients that can be treated in a day. You don't want to have more than you can handle, but you also don't want to have empty rooms. So it's a matter of finding that balance, and then leaving a little bit of leeway because patients will be late and other things will come up throughout the day that can create delays.

For example, if you are running an IV therapy clinic and you are scheduling a morbidly obese patient, there's a high likelihood that it might take more time to place that patient's IV. This could be a problem because you don't want your other patients to be waiting; you want everyone to have a good experience. In that case, you may want to book the more challenging IV insertion as the last patient of the day or leave extra time between this patient and the following appointment.

You could create a thirty-minute window instead of a ten-minute window between patients in case you have a "hard stick." It truly is the little things like these that matter. Each detail that is preemptively addressed greatly increases the odds that the patient will have a great experience and become your clinic's greatest fan.

Clinic Check-in

Clinic check-in is another aspect of your service that must be streamlined. This is a part of the patient experience that is critical. It's their first interaction with your clinic. It's important to have a smooth flow through your practice from the moment they set foot in your practice.

Ideally, when the patient comes in, they will have already filled out their pre-screening questionnaires electronically beforehand, but you should have clipboards with the paperwork ready to go. If you are charting electronically, then have a tablet or computer ready for them.

If they haven't filled the forms out online, you can quickly hand them what they need as soon as they walk in. Those forms then serve as a general check-in. They should include their pre-screening questionnaire, your privacy practice policy, and anything else that every patient would need to receive and sign for.

Consent forms can be given to them during the check-in to review or after the provider talks about it with them. However, it should only be signed by the patient *after* the provider has explained everything and answered questions.

It all boils down to making the experience of both parties (customer and whoever is attending to them) as smooth as possible. You don't want a situation where you get a patient in the waiting room and you give them one piece of paperwork to fill out, then ten minutes go by and you call them back over, waving a piece of paper in the air and saying, "Oh, I forgot to give you this one." That's not great service.

Great service is about anticipating needs, wants, and questions, then preemptively addressing them before the patient needs to even bring them up. Remember how my glass of iced tea at the Ritz Carlton was never more than half empty so I never had to wait for a refill? My server was a master at preemptively addressing my needs.

While the patient is filling out their forms, the front desk should already know which treatment rooms are available for the patient. The rooms should be prepared and sanitized every time. Walking a patient back to a dirty room should never happen. Yet it is something that has happened to me many times as a patient. That does *not* create a "wow" experience. I can't emphasize enough how all the little things add up to make the patient experience amazing.

I've been to medical offices where the check-in process almost seems to have been set up to intentionally make it difficult and inefficient. One time I went to see my insurance-based primary care provider. I signed in and then waited for over 30 minutes to even be acknowledged and provided with my check-in paperwork. It was another 30 minutes before I was placed in an exam room and an additional 45 minutes before the doctor even walked in. Horrendous.

This could have happened because they overbooked themselves or just because they don't have a good flow (or management) within their practice. It makes things chaotic and disorganized and generally ends with the patient having a miserable and frustrating experience.

Needless to say, I didn't ever return to that practice. Now I pay $69 a month for access to a Direct Primary Care office, where the service is outstanding and the wait time is always under 10 minutes.

To get a better feel for what the experience would be for your customer, you should run some live simulations prior to opening. Practice with employees, friends, or family, and do some role-playing.

They should enter the practice as if they are patients being moved through the clinic as if they are being treated. When you're going through these test runs, check them all in, one by one, and transfer them around your clinic the same way you would with a real patient. Move them into the exam rooms, and have a provider (or a person playing the role) come in to chat with them for five or ten minutes.

You could all pretend like it's a busy day and try to create scenarios of difficult situations that might come up. Make it fun by providing food and beverages at the end and be sure to get their honest feedback. Doing this is a great way to prevent or minimize potential problems or bad experiences that could be solved before opening day when the real patients start to come in.

Discharge and Checkout

Checkout is another aspect of your service that you will want to streamline. It is pretty straightforward. Some services and treatments require patient follow-up so it is important to schedule the next appointment or phone follow-up before they leave your practice.

Certainly, someone on the clinical staff should ensure that they are stable and document that the patients do not have any complaints or complications before they leave. You can't discharge a patient if they have more pain than usual after a treatment and then just tell them to get in their car and leave.

You have to be very meticulous about how your practice discharges your patients, how you assess them prior to discharge, and how you follow up with them.

Collecting Payments

There are a couple of different schools of thought on how to go about collecting payments. I recommend collecting your payment upfront if you're providing a self-pay service. You will *always* want to collect payments upfront if you're providing a service like ketamine therapy.

Perception is key, and even if pricing was clearly discussed ahead of time and agreed upon, administering a mind-altering substance and then collecting payment could be perceived negatively, so it is best to avoid those types of situations.

There are a variety of payment processing services that you can use. These are sometimes referred to as credit card merchant services. Some may also include point-of-sale software. Many new clinics keep it simple by using something like Square. Square is convenient to use, but they also charge a high credit card processing fee. Credit card processing fees are typically 2.5–3.2%.

If you prefer savings over simplicity, you can work with the bank where you opened your business account. They almost always have a credit card processing service that they offer. Sometimes the fees are lower, and you can often rent or buy a credit card machine.

There are additional merchant service providers out there, and we regularly update our training programs with some of the best options.

If you accept cash payments, you have a few additional details to iron out. Will you have a safe for cash? What type of safe and where will you put it? How much cash will you keep in your practice overnight? Who's going to take the deposits to the bank? Will you be making a deposit after dark? Or will you leave cash locked in your clinic until the next day? Think ahead, make a decision, and then write the policy and procedure on it.

Refunds

Refunds are a part of payment processing. A word of warning: there are going to be times when you might have delivered perfect service and care, but somebody is going to want a refund. It could be for any number of reasons. Rarely, it's nothing more than people trying to get things for free.

My wife was recently in a salon, and there was a lady there who had just gotten her nails done. The lady sat next to my wife the entire time and never told the person doing her nails that there was a problem or that she was doing something she didn't like. She was smiling and joking around with the person doing her

226 Clinic Launch Secrets

nails. After her nails were finished, and she reached the check-out counter, she complained that the nails were terrible and that she didn't want to pay for them. According to my wife, though, she seemed to love the work while it was being done, but her demeanor flipped as soon as it was time to pay.

Situations like that are very uncommon in the medical field, but occasionally you will have a patient or client who wants a refund or a discount. It can be very frustrating, but in most cases, for a self-pay clinic, it's best to just give them a refund. If you don't, there is a good chance they will head over to Google, Yelp, or the BBB and leave you a terrible review. It's not worth it.

Refund them. Follow the proper procedure to discharge the patient from the care of your clinic, and place them on the list of patients who are not welcome back.

Provider Evaluations

Providers evaluate patients. They look at the whole picture—their medical history as well as their chief complaint—and then create the treatment plan. Then they write any orders for treatments or medications. That's what should be done in every practice, even if you're just giving something as simple as a bag of fluids.

Running your practice without providers ever evaluating patients is dangerous. I've seen practices where there are no providers at all. Everything's just operated on a standing order or standing protocol. These practices often have a medical director who creates a standing order or standing protocol; they authorize RNs to treat patients without being properly evaluated. That is a malpractice lawsuit waiting to happen.

Providers are all trained that they need to evaluate patients prior to writing orders unless it is an emergency. If your providers practice the way they were trained, your clinic is going to be fine. You don't want to take shortcuts with something like blanket standing-orders or protocols. You'd be setting yourself up for major problems.

Provider evaluations are the standard of care. They ensure that the patient is getting treatments and/or medication that's appropriate for their current health status. Set up your system in such a way that everybody is seen by a provider at least once.

At that point, the provider can write standing orders and those standing orders can potentially be used for months—for as long as the clinic owner and the physician, or the provider, are comfortable with.

Always practice the way you were trained until you have a valid reason for changing. And no, convenience or cost saving is not a valid reason. I am talking about high-quality, peer-reviewed medical literature or a published standard of care change by an authoritative organization.

Follow-Up

Follow-up is another part of your practice that can be streamlined. In some cases, this could mean automating parts of it. There are two types of follow-ups: there's medical follow-up and customer service follow-up.

For the customer service follow-up, the best place to do it is in the clinic because you have their attention. The Federal Trade Commission (FTC) has strict rules on how reviews that are going to be made public for marketing can be collected and incentivized. If any remuneration is given to a patient for leaving a review, it must be disclosed, if it is used in marketing materials.

Remuneration could be something as small as a discount, a free service, or even a $10 Starbucks gift card. If a public review is incentivized, it must be disclosed. Now, if the review or feed-back is used for internal purposes only, there is no problem with incentivizing a patient for completing a review or feedback form. It's basically a reward to entice them to take a few minutes and fill out a survey, or whatever else you may use to assess feedback and improve the experience.

The Net Promoter Score (NP Score) is a simple and easy tool that can be used internally to assess patient satisfaction. The feedback would be in the form of a range of scores, from one to ten. If you get a low score, then you use follow-up questions to ask what the clinic could do better.

You could also ask one or two simple questions in the form of a survey via text messages. You could send them a specified amount of time after they leave the office, maybe an hour later. A cus-tomer relationship management (CRM) software tool can easily automate that for you.

Your response to online feedback can set you apart. Go to your reviews on Google or Yelp, or wherever you have your business listed, and make sure that you are following up with anybody and everybody who left a review.

It is very important to leave a professional response to any nega-tive reviews. How a business owner responds to a negative review can say more about the business than one hundred 5-star reviews. Don't miss the opportunity to apologize and demonstrate publicly that your customers matter and that you will professionally correct the situation.

Get feedback in whatever form you can. This data matters. Then you can take that data and graph it so you can see trends. I'd even put it on display during meetings or in a break room so everyone is aware that you are paying attention and striving to make improvements.

CHAPTER SIXTEEN

THE EXPLOSIVE POWER OF MARKETING

*"The real fact of the matter is that nobody reads ads.
People read what interests them,
and sometimes it's an ad."*

—Howard Luck Gossage

When I got started as a clinic owner, I had never built a "real" business before, and I didn't know much about marketing or patient acquisition. Before then, my only business experience was working for a chain restaurant and a couple of small side hustles.

And let me tell you, managing an IHOP or a Macaroni Grill was a *lot* different from starting and operating my own clinic from scratch. In chain restaurants, the corporation tells management exactly what to do, creates all the policies and procedures, tells you exactly where to order every supply from, sets your prices, and handles all the marketing and customer acquisition.

When I managed the restaurants, customers would simply come in when they were hungry. It was simply my job to ensure the operation ran according to the blueprint so that customers received consistent meals quickly. With that type of system in place, I never even thought about marketing.

When I was planning my business, I had no idea where to start with marketing. The reality is, marketing a medical practice is very simple. In most areas, there are more patients looking for self-pay clinic services than there are clinics to handle them, so all you need to do is make it easy for patients to find you.

Marketing is the number one business skill that every entrepreneur *must* study and understand. Sure you can outsource to an agency, but nearly all operated the same way. I worked with several before I decided to learn the skill myself and in-house all our marketing efforts.

First and foremost, no agency will care more about your business, or market your business with more passion, than you will. Agencies are notorious for starting off strong, accepting more clients than they can handle, and then generating lackluster results. Most agencies will only put in the amount of effort required to retain a customer or prevent them from complaining, nothing more. There is a rare breed of agency that charges for results only, but those are few and far between. Head on over to **jasonduprat.com/book** to learn about our results-focused and results-guaranteed marketing services.

People need to know that your business exists and how it can help them, period. You could have the best product or service in the world, but if no one knows about it, then it doesn't matter. You won't be able to generate enough sales to succeed.

If you want to boost your odds of success, then you must become a master of marketing or you must have someone on your team who will fill that role. Trust me, if you can complete years of college, pass licensing exams, and provide great care to complex patients, then you are more than capable of learning how to be a great marketer. I could write an entire book on how to successfully market your clinic, but here I will just touch on the very basics needed to get started.

Oh, and before the thought crosses your mind, do not even consider getting a degree in marketing. College teaches outdated and ineffective marketing content and strategies. This is especially true when it comes to digital marketing.

Digital marketing simply changes too fast for college professors to keep up. Professors are too busy conducting research, politicking, and teaching from the power points that the textbooks provide. The overwhelming majority of professors who teach digital marketing have no technical, in-the-trenches marketing skills. They simply regurgitate outdated approaches that are usually at least three to four years old by the time it hits their classroom.

Marketing—especially digital marketing—is best learned from those who are doing it every day. Those in the trenches are masters at setting up and using sophisticated tracking software, they work diligently to perfect their sales copy, they write email nurture sequences daily, they understand the metrics and KPIs, and they know how to track and measure the return on their marketing dollars.

I guarantee you won't learn any of that practical real-world information from 99% of college marketing instructors. Sorry, you just won't, it changes too fast and great marketers can earn 3–4x what a college can afford to pay a professor.

College is good for some degrees, but it is terrible at providing quality education on some topics. Digital marketing is one of those, so sign up for a course from an actual marketer and start immediately implementing what you learn. There is no better way to get really good at something than by learning from someone great and then putting in the reps needed to achieve excellence.

We can cover some marketing basics here but we don't want to get too into the weeds. As I said, the details change with evolving technologies and many technologies evolve fast. There are some important things to think about very early on. These include your marketing funnel, plan, your patient avatar, your marketing campaigns, marketing tools, and more.

Your Marketing Plan

Your marketing plan starts with knowing exactly who your ideal patient is. These are the people you want to attract, so develop your marketing plan around them. Many practices fall into the trap of trying to attract nearly *every* type of patient.

The ones who fail end up offering 15 or 20 unrelated services without being great at delivering or marketing any one of them. This doesn't make a lot of sense. It is a classic example of how new entrepreneurs often lack clarity and goals in their business. They are merely chasing the dollars instead of taking the time to assess who their ideal client is, what service they are most interested in providing, and what it is that they are passionate about.

Having a new practice where you have 15 or 20 different services is challenging because you will have to market all of those services in addition to performing them. It is much easier to start with a specialized niche because you have only one patient avatar, which will serve as the main type of patient that you are trying to attract. As you grow, you can always add on complementary services, but only do it when your patients start asking for them.

If you have a specialty practice, niche down and focus on marketing 1–2 services to start. A Med Spa may offer a variety of aesthetic services and procedures, but if they are especially great at performing non-invasive body sculpting procedures then this is the best place to start when it comes to their marketing.

Once you identify your ideal patient, then you are in the best position to speak to their exact pain points. This is a crucial step. Get into the mind of your customer to find out what their struggles are.

What do they think about at night while they're lying in bed? If you want to be good at marketing, you have to be able to put yourself in the shoes of the person you're trying to market to. You have to become a master of empathy. Figure out exactly what they're going through, what stresses them out, and what makes them unhappy. Then, intertwine those words, thoughts, and emotions into your marketing materials.

Marketing is simply helping people understand that your product or service can help them move from the island of pain to the island of pleasure. People pay for products and services because they have some sort of problem and they want a solution. If the value of the solution exceeds the cost associated with their problem then they will make the investment.

I have noticed that the best marketers and clinicians are those who have struggled personally with something for which they are offering a solution. They naturally know exactly what a patient is going through so they can craft a message that resonates with their ideal patient—because their ideal patient used to be them!

In the aesthetics world, the pain point could be something physical that they dislike about themselves. It could be something that detracts from their self-confidence or something that they try to cover up or hide. It could be as trivial as a wrinkle or something bigger such as severe facial acne.

If you are providing ketamine therapy for treatment-resistant depression you could describe how feeling depressed all the time can lead to a downward spiral. Feeling down makes it hard to get pleasure from hobbies or sports or other activities that maybe they used to enjoy. Maybe that lack of joy has caused them to self-medicate with food or alcohol. Too much food could have caused them to gain weight, which in turn worsened their self-confidence and triggered a deeper depression. Or maybe the alcohol has caused them health problems or resulted in relationship problems. Whatever their situation is, you must be able to empathetically embody what they experience and what they feel.

If you can pinpoint the exact thoughts and emotions they go through as a result of their condition or problem, you can quickly capture their attention and present your treatment (the solution to their condition or problem). Doing this with compassion for their struggles lets them know you understand how they feel and what they are going through. This is the only way that you can relate to potential patients and let them know that you understand and can help them. If your product or service can truly help them, you have a moral obligation to bring it to their attention.

Your Marketing Pitch

When talking to clients or others in the community about what your clinic does, you need a simple short marketing pitch. It should be no more than a sentence or two.

The purpose of the pitch isn't to get others to become your customer instantly or to immediately adopt your idea. The purpose is to craft a compelling statement that fosters the start of a conversation.

This is often referred to as your elevator pitch. It should be able to describe your service or clinic if you only had a short elevator ride in which to do it. It should describe what your clinic does or who it helps, it should include a description of the result, and allude to how you do it.

A good marketing pitch for a ketamine clinic owner might be: "We provide symptom relief for patients suffering from treatment-resistant depression with ketamine therapy."

These are created as very simple statements for a reason. You want everyone to easily understand exactly who you serve and what you do. A great marketing pitch creates curiosity. For example, "Isn't ketamine a horse tranquilizer?" or "What's treatment-resistant depression?" or "How much ketamine is administered?" Curiosity built. Conversation started. Now rapport can be developed. It's that simple.

I couldn't tell you the number of conferences I have been to where I ask someone to tell me what they do in their business and they spend 10 minutes and an enormous amount of mental energy trying to explain it. Keeping it concise can sometimes be a challenge for healthcare professionals. We tend to have a lot of information stored in our minds and can sometimes fall into the trap of attempting to demonstrate how much we know.

Keep it simple and short or you will see eyes glaze over as those you are talking to try to figure out how to exit the conversation. Believe me when I say—no patient cares about you, your business, or what you know. They only care about what you can do for them.

Pre-Launch Marketing

Pre-launch marketing is often what will give your clinic the momentum it needs to grow quickly in the first several months after opening. Pre-clinic marketing should commence at least 3–4 months before you open.

First, get a website built and get your clinic on Google Maps as soon as you have a confirmed location. This will ensure that people can find you locally. The website should be capable of booking appointments, explaining the services that you offer, and should include your hours of operation as well as your antici-pated grand-opening date.

If you aren't fortunate enough to get some attention from the local media outlets, then you will find that most of the patients who will find your clinic when you first open will do so through Google search. With a Google Maps presence, it will be easy for people to find directions to your practice. These two things are mandatory. You have close to a 100% chance of failing if you do not have a website that shows up on a Google search or if you are not on Google maps.

You need to join and get involved with your local Chamber of Commerce; this is a key part of having a successful brick-and-mortar business. Not only will it build up your connection with others in the community but they often share information about different business resources that could help your clinic succeed.

Municipalities and area leadership love new businesses coming into town because it brings jobs and growth. The more you can get in front of people who support small businesses, the better.

I've seen a lot of clinics that have done their PR really well. They work with their local organizations, and I've even seen mayors attend a small clinic's ribbon-cutting ceremony. Politicians love to showcase economic growth, and it'll often make news if they show up. Free marketing from the local press is one of the best types of marketing a new business can receive.

Another pre-launch marketing strategy that works well is work-ing with publicists to write press releases about your grand opening, special discounts for military, charitable work, or other social causes that your clinic is helping. This type of PR can be particularly effective, especially if a local news station decides to pick up the story and air it. Even if they don't, the backlinks to your website that are created when online media outlets publish your press release can help boost your clinic's Google search rankings.

A detailed breakdown of pre-launch marketing is outside the scope of this book, but you should be aware of other marketing efforts such as direct mail, clinic fliers, and other types of campaigns to let people know that you're about to open.

When you start marketing ahead of time and can accept patient appointments on your website, there is no reason you shouldn't have at least 25–50 appointments booked before you open.

The biggest marketing mistake I've seen a lot of people make is that they do absolutely no marketing until after they open their doors. It's unfortunate. They quickly find themselves sitting in an empty clinic with nothing to do for several weeks. Talk about a morale killer. In business, you want to have momentum on your side. Start marketing early and build up that momentum.

You want to hit the ground running—with patients already booked when you open. Even before you open up shop, you will want to invest in paid marketing. For example, you could put an ad in your local paper or set up local digital ads.

There are many forms of paid marketing. At a minimum, I would suggest setting aside at least $3,000 to cover your pre-opening marketing. You can't rely on word of mouth and more organic forms of marketing until you create a horde of raving fans for your clinic.

Your Marketing Campaign

There are a variety of different strategies you could use in carrying out your marketing campaign. Every clinic is different in terms of what type of campaign will work best for them, but your strategy should include paid marketing and non-paid marketing. With paid marketing, there is typically a bit of trial and error needed to determine where your best ROI will come from.

Some elements of your marketing campaign might include:

Email Marketing Campaign

An email campaign is something every clinic should have for both leads and patient engagement. You can set up contact creation and email collection through your customer relationship management (CRM) software or an email service provider. Today these tools have started to become one and the same.

If a patient books an appointment or interacts with some piece of marketing material that you have (such as your website or a lead magnet), it is important to collect their contact information. A more advanced marketer would also add more detail to the contacts on their email list by adding tags that indicate which types of products or services they are interested in.

If a prospective patient clicks a link to your clinic's Botox page and then downloads a Botox PDF, obviously that client should be tagged as a lead that is interested in Botox. This is called segregating your audience. You can then send them a fairly short automated email sequence that is educational and specifically addresses the common questions and concerns that a Botox patient might have. Structure it to have five or six emails that get sent out twice a week for a few weeks.

That type of email campaign is also called an email nurture sequence. These allow you to put yourself in front of your contact constantly, letting them know who you are and how you can serve them. If what you are sending them is just a sales pitch or high-pressure, book-now emails, they will unsubscribe, so don't do it.

The key here is to provide value in your emails and the easiest way to do that is to provide free education. It has to be something that's helpful and important to them. It should speak their exact language and talk to their exact pain points. This is why segregating your email list is critical.

You can create nurture sequences for your top products and services and send them to those you know are wanting to learn more because they clicked a link or downloaded a resource that indicated they are interested in a specific service. If you execute this properly, you will get their attention immediately because your email copy was speaking directly to their pain points and questions. I have built an incredibly powerful CRM software that is pre-loaded with proven email nurture sequences. It also simplifies patient scheduling, texting, and appointment reminders to take all the guesswork out of your marketing and patient follow-up. To learn more visit: jasonduprat.com/LeadFuel

Traditional Marketing Tools

Billboards

A billboard can also serve as a means of marketing. You can set up something small and inexpensive like the ones you see on sidewalk benches. Those are some of the lowest-cost billboards.

Then there are those gigantic billboards on the highway. The cost of those billboards can be astronomical, but they get a lot of eyes on them. Are they the right eyes though? Billboards are not very targeted. In most cases, only a tiny fraction of everybody who sees one is a potential customer. That is why you typically see large healthcare systems, banks, and attorneys paying for that space. They often have a very broad customer base.

Billboards may not be the best marketing strategy for a specialized clinic because not everybody is in the market for niche services such as eyelash extensions, IV infusions, or ketamine therapy. If you had a generic primary care service or something not very specialized that most people could use, then maybe it would work. Otherwise, it would be hard to justify the expense of paying for views from those who do not fit within the mold of your ideal patient avatar.

The companies that sell billboard space track the amount of traffic that occurs where it is placed and they use that to set their prices. So, let's say 10,000 cars drive by the billboard every day and there is an average of 1.25 people in each car. The company would then charge for 12,500 impressions or views.

Now, we all know that drivers and passengers are not eagerly staring out their windows to see every billboard, so in reality, only a small percentage of those 12,500 people driving by would even see the billboard, let alone read it. I personally think billboards are way overpriced. They are better leveraged as a vanity marketing tool or just for general brand awareness for large companies.

Television

Television can also be a means of marketing. You can leverage TV ads, but those are pretty expensive. One affordable option that is great for clinics and small businesses is running on the morning show segment; most larger cities offer this. In New Mexico for example, there is a morning news show called *Good Day New Mexico*. Almost every city has its own version of these. They usually set it up to look like an actual news show with a TV interview.

Essentially, you, as the practice owner (or whoever is representing you) apply and pay to be interviewed on their morning show. You now have the chance to talk about your business and your products on TV.

You'll typically give them a list of questions beforehand, then when you show up on set they have everything ready for you. You just chat with the host during the amount of time allotted for the spot you paid for. They will ask you questions based on your business and the patients that you serve.

In the process, you'll want to deliver value and information about a condition, service, or disease process, while also putting yourself out there as the expert in whatever treatment that you offer. Then they give you a video clip that you have the rights to and can edit into smaller clips that you can repurpose for content on your website and social media platforms.

This is something worth looking into as it's generally a good value. You can leverage that interview to build credibility. After all, you were just on the set of a local TV channel and interviewed by a familiar and trustworthy face from the news station. It could be a pretty good deal in my opinion. Using this type of TV advertisement is an effective and inexpensive way to go for a start-up clinic, but it is also not very targeted.

Other types of paid TV ads will be a bit more targeted. Advertising companies can get your TV commercials in front of a targeted audience by airing them on a specific channel and during a specific show, and you will choose a channel to air based on the demographics of that channel or a show's audience. For instance, if you offer a service to the elderly population, you might use a channel that plays reruns of the TV shows they loved when they were younger.

Radio

Radio ads are another paid marketing option. You probably won't want to test them until you have opened your practice. Radio ads, again, are not ultra-targeted. From my own experience, I don't think a lot of people actually listen to them.

Radio listenership is declining, and whenever I hear a radio commercial, most of the time I tune it out or change the station. I just don't think radio ads are very valuable. We tested them once and lost thousands of dollars because they didn't generate a single patient. We only got one lead that led to one phone call. The person didn't even show up for their booked appointment.

Radio just didn't work for us, but they have worked for others, so don't completely rule it out. Based on the market we were in and the station we chose, I am not a fan. Pick the station your ideal patient avatar would most likely be listening to.

Direct Mail

For this direct mail advertising, you would mail a postcard, flier, or letter directly to a potential patient or to providers for referrals. We loved this strategy. We paid a freelancer to collect the addresses of potential referring providers for us and created a postcard to let them know we were in town and accepting referrals.

When you are calculating costs, include things such as the cost of building your mailing list. That's a fixed expense. You also have to know how much you'll pay to mail out each postcard. Factor in the size of the postcard, the weight of the stock you print it on, and whether you want a glossy or matte finish. Don't forget about postage costs, either.

If you'll be using direct mail, commit to doing it for at least four to six months. If you only send them out once, you will likely receive only a small number of responses. The key element for direct mail success is to be consistent with your touches (a marketing touchpoint is a distinct point of contact you have with a potential patient or client).

Your market should always get a similar piece of mail at regular intervals. If a provider sees the same postcard saying that you accept referrals on their desk over and over again, there is a much higher probability of them reaching out to learn more or sending a patient your way.

Digital Marketing Tools

Websites

A good website will help prospective patients find you quickly. You don't have to have a ton of information on the site at first. Place some information about who your practice serves on the home page and create an "About Us" section where you describe more about your practice and why you chose to start it.

You could also include some information on the providers who work in the clinic, what the patient can expect, and some frequently asked questions. It's a good idea to have details about who you treat and what your payment model is. If it is self-pay only and you don't take insurance, make that very clear.

The more thorough the information on your website is, the less time you will squander answering generic inquiries. As a new business owner, reducing the time you spend on the phone is a small but effective way to maximize your clinic's productivity.

When it comes to building your clinic's website there are a couple of options:

Build Your Own

If you are mildly tech-savvy and a do-it-yourselfer, you can create your own website and easily save $1,000 to $2,000. If you're not technically inclined, this is probably not something you want to attempt on your own.

The ease of use of many online website creation tools is truly amazing. The best website creation platforms are no more difficult to use than your typical word-processing application. In fact, these days, you can create a website with zero coding knowledge using easy-to-use drag-and-drop website editors.

I personally use Wix, but there are many other options out there. I think Wix is a great option because it is easy to use. It has an SEO Wizard that helps you scan your site for the most important areas that might be suboptimal as it relates to SEO. The tool tells you exactly how to fix each SEO deficiency. Squarespace is also another web-building tool that we used when we first built our podcasting website. In my opinion, it is not as user-friendly as Wix, but it still does the job.

Another advantage of building your website yourself is that you will maintain complete control over the look, design, and access. Since you created the website, it will be easy to update without having to involve anyone else. As things progress, if you need to make a change or add promotional information, you won't need to wait for your website developer to make the changes. Sometimes waiting on a third party for all the little website tweaks slows things down drastically.

Pay a Website Developer

If you decide to go this route, you can find a website developer online or locally. You can find web developers on freelancing sites such as Upwork or Fiverr or through references and referrals. The work that they have to do is pretty minimal because you are still going to have to provide them with all the images, website copy, pages, and menu links.

Website developers are not medical professionals, so they won't go and do research to properly describe the services and treatments provided in your clinic. Even if they did, you wouldn't want them to. You have a professional obligation to provide them with that information and to ensure everything on your website is accurate.

Since you will have to do all the heavy lifting when it comes to creating a website for your clinic, I usually recommend you handle the site buildout yourself if at all possible. There are now amazing templates that have 80% of the website build done for you.

You should use images of your *actual practice* and *team* (even if it's just you) on your website. Loading your website up with generic stock images is detrimental to building rapport with potential patients.

Most web developers will build the site for you and then provide you with administrative (admin) access. This admin access, among other things, allows you to log in and create new pages, make blog posts, edit text and add or update photos or videos. It is highly advisable to create the admin account yourself and then create a subaccount for the developer. This ensures that you retain ownership and total control of the website.

If a fly-by-night online web developer creates your admin account when building your site and later disappears after they are paid, you may have an extremely difficult time gaining ownership of (or administrative access to) the site.

You should also always buy the domain name yourself from a domain name registrar such as Namecheap. Never let anyone else buy, own, or otherwise control your domain name or website.

If you choose to have a developer create your website, make sure you obtain a signed contract stating that you own everything they create on your behalf. You must own the actual site, the domain name, any content they create, the design, and access to the main admin account.

Google Business and Google Maps

Google Business and Google Maps are completely free marketing. In today's day and age, if you do not have your business displaying on Google Maps, you are way behind the eight ball. You should definitely take advantage of having a free Google Business profile with your logo, operating hours, and phone number.

When you are setting up your Google Business account, they will ask you for your clinic's physical address. Google then sends a postcard to that address with a special code on it. That is how they will *verify* that your business exists at the address you provided. Without an actual location, they won't verify your Google Business profile. In this case, you will have to wait until you sign a lease and can receive mail before you can set one up.

Once you get verified, your clinic shows up on Google Maps almost immediately. You can and should update your Google Business profile as you progress with your clinic launch. If you don't have a business phone number, you could use a VOIP number or Google Voice phone number to get started. Always make sure that your information is up to date because a lot of patients will use Google Maps as a way to discover and locate your clinic.

Adding posts is another part of leveraging the Google Business platform. Google will even try to encourage you to do so by sending you email reminders. If somebody in your area is searching for your clinic services, some keywords in your post could help them easily locate you. Posts are considered relevant for about two weeks, and then you'll have to update them.

You can also leverage your Google Business profile to share promos and other marketing content. If you post your promotions or discounts be sure to remove them when the offer is no longer available or you will get calls and emails weeks later with patients asking to get the promotional price.

Paid Advertisements

Paid ads are another important tool for marketing. Most niche self-pay practices need to be very targeted. Along with every single other piece of marketing you create, your paid ads should have calls-to-action (CTAs). It can be as obvious as "Schedule a Free Consultation" or it can be a more subtle invitation, "Find Out More." It could instruct them to "Fill out an assessment," or it could tell the viewer to "Click the link" and download a free PDF file or ebook.

You can even run promotional ads offering a discount on your services, in exchange for their name, email, and phone number that say something like, "We have a coupon, and if you want 30% off our service, enter your name and email address, and we'll email you the coupon."

When it comes to paid marketing, the one thing that separates the amateurs from the pros is their ability to track the leads generated and accurately calculate their Return on Ad Spend (ROAS). ROAS = Gross Sales from Paid Ads / Cost of Paid Ads.

If you can fine-tune your paid ads so that they are able to produce $5+ in revenue for each dollar spent on paid ads, then you have just created a marketing ATM that pumps money out. The best clinic owners test and optimize their paid marketing until they hit similar or better metrics. At that point, it is just a matter of pumping more money into the marketing engine.

When done properly, more money invested into paid ads results in predictable revenue generation. For those willing to learn and master the skills of marketing, the payoff can be tremendous.

I could write an entire book on the topic of paid marketing. I absolutely love it, and there is a lot to learn. It will likely become a major component of a future book or training program because so many healthcare professionals erroneously perceive marketing as an expense versus an investment. They simply don't understand the concept of tracking their marketing efforts. They don't understand that investing $1 in paid advertising can easily result in $5 or more in immediate gross revenue for the clinic.

If they were to then factor in how much each patient spends at their clinic over their lifetime, (something called Customer Lifetime Value or CLV), they could see the ROI from a paid ad that helps them acquire a single new patient might be as high as 10x, 20x, or even more!

It's all about mastering marketing concepts and the relevant metrics associated with paid marketing. Once those skills are obtained, it's a game changer because most, if not all, of your competitors won't take the time to learn them. Dan Kennedy once said, "The business that can afford to spend the most to acquire a customer wins."

There is a lot to unpack before a business can know how much it can profitably spend to acquire a new patient. The truth is 99% of clinic owners simply don't know how much they can spend to attract a new patient, so they end up investing little to nothing on their paid marketing efforts. But you, my friend, you read this book. If you master these marketing concepts above and know your marketing numbers, you will have the upper hand on all your competitors who haven't mastered these concepts.

Social Media

Social media marketing is the process of gaining traffic or attention for a product or service by leveraging social media platforms. Your practice must have a strong online presence for patients and providers to be able to discover your clinic. Creating social media accounts for your practice on various social media platforms is one of the easiest places to start. You can then start making frequent posts to those platforms. Constant and consistent engagement with potential patients is important in social media marketing.

To set up your social media presence, you should create accounts on the following platforms (listed in the order of priority):

- YouTube
- Facebook
- Instagram
- LinkedIn

I recommend creating business profiles on all of these platforms. These profiles should have links to your clinic's website and provide other relevant information.

When it comes to consistently creating and posting content for your clinic, I would recommend starting with a single platform. Once you are familiar with it and have established the account, you can move on to the next and start building your business presence there.

Using this step-by-step approach, you don't get overwhelmed with learning all the social media platforms at once and struggling to keep up with them. Once you are ready to post on other platforms, you can speed up the process by using a social media management software that will post to multiple social media accounts on various platforms all at the same time or they can even be pre-scheduled to post on a specific day or time.

Social media is social. People are not coming onto most social media platforms hoping to see a new ad from your business about its latest special achievement or update. They're on social media to be entertained, they want to see what their friends and family are up to, check out pictures of cute animals, or see people doing weird or funny things. People will not care about you or your business until there is something in it for them.

Adopt a personality that fits your brand and the social media platform you're posting on and make your content valuable, interesting, and engaging so that viewers are getting what they want. Simply make your content informational and related to the services your clinic offers.

YouTube

YouTube is great. If it were me starting up a new clinic, I would start by producing videos and posting them on YouTube. It is a perfect platform for creating educational content. When you upload YouTube videos, make sure you tag them with relevant keywords that potential patients might be searching for that also relate to the video's content.

If the video you create is aiming to get referring providers to watch it, then use keywords that a provider might be searching for. Your tags and videos should always include information about your location (city and state), so your video pops up on a local search.

A lot of patients found me and my practice on YouTube because of the handful of educational and patient experience videos I uploaded to the clinic's channel. I even had patients flying in from other states to come to my practice because they had watched the YouTube videos that I made.

When a patient watches you on video, they perceive a rapport already being developed. They see your face and watch your demeanor and professional behavior. If your content is quality they will see that you are knowledgeable.

When these things all fall into place, they start to feel as though they know you, they might start to like you, and they may even trust you, all before ever meeting you. This is the power of video.

Additionally, videos on YouTube do not go anywhere. They are searchable and can be found years after you have made them.

That creates more leverage when compared to social media platforms such as Facebook, where your content will only show up for a limited amount of time, typically for as long as it is getting a substantial amount of engagement (likes, comments, and shares). Then, once the algorithm determines that it is not worth showing, it disappears into the social media ether, likely never to be seen again.

If you're going to do videos, even if you are primarily planning to create them for a different social media platform, I highly recommend putting them on YouTube. They're searchable forever, not to mention YouTube is the number two most used search engine in the world.

LinkedIn

LinkedIn is good, but I don't think it's the best place to be marketing a medical clinic—unless you're primarily marketing for referrals. I see people on LinkedIn making posts targeting patients, but LinkedIn is not designed for that.

LinkedIn is a professional networking platform. If you intend to network with a provider in hopes of earning future referrals, this is the platform to use. In that case, your posts should be geared toward educating and getting those referrals from other healthcare practitioners.

If your intention is to market directly to patients, LinkedIn isn't the best place. Their ads cost substantially more and Linkedin isn't the place where you see ads for private clinics. There are always exceptions to every rule, but in most cases, the content you post there should be aimed at educating local providers and building relationships with them so they feel confident referring patients to you.

Facebook

Your clinic's presence on Facebook should consist of a Facebook business page. Marketing your business on your personal profile can work, but for a healthcare professional, it is not the best way.

As a clinic owner, you really don't want your patients seeing you toasting that glass of wine or lying on the beach in your man thongs. The goal is not to become a social media influencer; it is to generate leads and sales for your clinic. Don't get it confused or fall into the trap of trying to gain followers and likes. Those are vanity metrics that mean nothing for your business.

You want to foster leads and nurture new patients. The strategy is very different from the strategy of becoming an influencer. Instead, you should create a new business profile, and then anything that has to do with your business should be shared from that page.

You can then use your personal profile to refer people back to your business page. That's the most professional way to market your business on Facebook. Messages and posts related to your clinic should all be coming from your business page.

Encourage your patients and those who match your ideal patient avatar to like and follow your page. Do not ask all your friends and relatives from all over the country and the world to like your page, it doesn't matter. They are not your ideal patients.

You want people who are patients or who closely resemble your ideal patient to follow your page. That way, they get notifications when you make posts and they are much more likely to engage with your posts because they are relevant to them and their interests. This tells the algorithms to continue showing the post to more page followers.

If you do it right, it will help you establish your online social media presence. Don't forget that this is not a numbers game. The quality of your followers and those who like your page is far more important than the quantity.

Having a business page is a great way to start getting your clinic out there. It is one more digital location that can be found by potential patients or other providers who might refer patients to you. Try to make at least two to three posts on your business page every week. Consistency is key.

Paid Facebook Advertising

We discussed paid ads previously, but there are a few special things to know as it relates to paid ads on Facebook. First, Facebook has gotten much more strict on enforcing its advertising policies, and it is very important to follow their policies.

Running the wrong ads that violate policies will cause the algorithm to automatically reject the ad, and if you try to run too many ads that violate policies, the ad account might get closed permanently. Even if that does happen, it isn't the end of the world because you can make a new account, but you'll have to start all over again.

Once you understand the advertising rules, you can create very targeted ads that are directed toward very specific geographical locations, user age, and user interests. This helps you put very specific ads in front of very specific people. It can be highly cost-effective when you know what you're doing.

Just like your YouTube videos, make sure that your social media posts and ads are not just sales pitches. They should be adding value. Educate the patients and the public about your products or services. Aim to provide free information that is entertaining and engaging.

Marketing Funnels

It took me years to learn, understand, and get good at marketing. In this section, I will run you through a crash course in marketing funnels. I will be throwing out some marketing terms without defining them. If they are new to you, ask Google or ChatGPT.

Marketing funnels are methods used to systematically move potential customers from hardly knowing your clinic exists to becoming paying patients. I am a visual learner, so let me paint the picture.

Imagine a funnel, the kind used to add oil to your vehicle—or, if you're a baker, to quickly transfer flour from a large jar to a much smaller one. At the very top of the funnel are your potential customers, which are also called leads.

(Honestly, I hate calling a patient a lead because to me that sounds so cold and robotic but for the sake of introducing you to the proper marketing terminology, I will stick with it.)

A lead must work his/her way down the funnel to the narrow bottom to become a patient. The funnel is smaller at the bottom because only a small percentage of patients that enter the funnel will become paying customers.

Now, imagine your clinic is sitting under the funnel, waiting to provide care for the paying patients as they come through the bottom of the funnel.

I like to use the marketing framework AIDA; this stands for Awareness, Interest, Desire, and Action. The purpose of a funnel is to move potential customers through these stages. Sometimes they can happen one step at a time, or you may be able to move them through multiple stages in a single interaction.

The first step is *awareness*. If a potential customer has never heard of your clinic before, they are referred to as a cold lead. This is because they are the hardest to sell something to. After all, they don't know your business at all. They certainly don't know how awesome you are. But as you publish marketing content, there will be a number of leads who become aware of your clinic and the services it provides.

Marketing material that engages a customer for the first time is always building awareness. Once a lead becomes aware of your business and starts to learn about the services you provide, some will start to gain *interest* and want to keep learning more.

Once they have an interest, you have accomplished step two and those who are interested will be eager to stay in touch and learn even more. This is where you can help them learn more about your clinic, the staff, and the services offered. This potential customer has moved from being part of a cold lead to a warm lead because they are two steps into the AIDA framework and halfway down the funnel.

As this person further engages with your marketing materials they begin to *desire* your service (aka the solution to a problem they have). Once they *desire* your product or service, you have accomplished step three. They are now even further down the funnel.

Typically, the more they engage with your business and the further along the AIDA framework they are, the warmer the lead becomes until eventually, right before they purchase, they are a hot lead.

An example of a hot lead might be someone who is trying to call your clinic to book an appointment. Or maybe you sell supplements on your clinic website. In that case, a hot lead would be a customer who made it to the checkout page and is ready to enter their credit card information to purchase.

Something that new clinic owners miss is the importance of capturing their lead's information so they can follow up. You must collect their email, name, and possibly a phone number, ideally on the first interaction.

The best way to collect their data is to offer something in exchange for sharing it. This could be a discount, a special offer, a free resource, a tool, or a helpful guide. In marketing, they have a variety of names for this, but let's call it a lead magnet.

Collecting the names and contact information of your potential clients so that you can continue to nurture them through the

AIDA framework via email is critical. After all, if you use paid ads to attract the lead to your lead magnet, you need to ensure you have a great follow-up email campaign in place. If you fail to follow up, that lead will be lost forever, and so will the money you spent to get them that far into the funnel.

As leads move from the top of the funnel to the bottom, you are essentially sorting out the people who aren't interested in coming into your clinic from the people who will. If you have "holes" in your funnel (not collecting contact information or failing to set up abandoned cart follow-up), then your marketing funnel will leak.

A leaky funnel is not generating all the patient appointments that it can and should. In other words, a leaky funnel is allowing for lost revenue. I don't want to get in the weeds with funnel optimization strategies here, but I do want you to be familiar with some marketing concepts including funnel optimization and leaky funnels.

When you are marketing, especially on social media, it all starts with the headline and the creative. The creative is the visual image or video that goes along with the social media post or paid ad. These elements are key because users on SM platforms are scanning before they decide if they want to read more.

Your headline and creative are going to be your very first impression. Your very first sentence on a written ad or post and the first few words on a video is what is called the *hook* in the marketing world. You want to *hook* the reader or viewer with something that catches their attention and lets them know the post is directly related to them. Then they will watch the rest of that video or read the rest of that post.

New clinic owners also tend to want instant results from paid ads. This is possible, but a greater percentage of sales typically come from the follow-up email nurture sequence.

Old data suggested that an average customer would need to see seven marketing messages (*touch points*) from a business before they purchase. These days, newer data suggests that the touch points could be as many as twenty-seven.

Multiple touch points over time help you develop rapport and trust with these potential patients. Sometimes, those come from paid ads, but the rest may come from your email nurture sequence, their phone calls to the clinic to ask a question, and their consultation with the provider before they know, like, and trust your clinic enough to make that decision to become your patient. Don't get discouraged if you run paid ads and don't get a flood of new patients instantly, that simply isn't how it works most of the time.

Nurture your leads. That's what it's all about. You send them emails or videos that demonstrate that you understand them and their pain points, you know what you're doing, and you know how to help them.

This is also where testimonials come into play. You should be asking every current or past patient who had a good experience for reviews and video testimonials. These should be included in your email nurture sequences, posted on social media, and added to your website.

Here is a teaser for those who like more advanced or techy strategies: you can leverage the Facebook pixel code by placing it on your website and then display ads specifically to those who viewed a certain page on the website. This is called *retargeting*.

One strategy is to *retarget* hot leads who were on the "Book an Appointment" page of your website with a video that invites them to a call because they likely just have one tiny objection or question that can easily be answered.

If you want to get fancy, you could also alternate what they see by *retargeting* them with testimonial videos from past patients. These ads will be displayed as they scroll through their Facebook newsfeed.

Your creativity and willingness to learn are the only real limits when it comes to leveraging digital marketing strategies to grow your clinic. Those who learn what it takes to be able to profitably spend the most to acquire their patients will, by default, become the leaders in their markets.

We cover clinic marketing in greater detail in our training programs. To learn more, visit:

jasonduprat.com/book

CHAPTER SEVENTEEN

GETTING OUT THERE: STAKE YOUR CLAIM

"The best way to find yourself is to lose yourself in the service of others."

—*Mahatma Gandhi*

There is a lot that goes into starting a clinic, and there are many really important things that I wish I knew before I started out. With that in mind, I would like to leave you with two final pieces of advice:

- Never be afraid to ask for help.
- Always learn from those who have accomplished what you want to accomplish.

The only reason I've achieved the success I have, is because I sought out those who were, where I wanted to be and asked for assistance. In many cases, I've compensated them for their time and ability to speed up my results. Whenever a problem comes up in my business that I'm struggling with, I look for someone who has already overcome similar problems, and I get their advice even if it costs me.

Why?

Because it's far faster and costs far less to ask your questions to someone who already has the answers rather than trying to figure them out for yourself. Doing this has saved me an untold number of hours and countless amounts of money.

If you are reading this book, you are already on the right track. You are doing some basic self-education. You are learning the steps and the methodologies that work. The fastest way to be successful is to replicate what has already proven to work and build upon that.

When I attended a mastermind with my mentor John Lee Dumas, who is the host of the top Entrepreneurship podcast in the world, he shared two important things:

1. He taught me about the importance of leveraging momentum in growing a business.

2. He also told me to never forget the Jim Rohn quote, "You are the average of the five people you spend the most time with."

He said that the quickest road to success is to spend more time with other successful business people. Not just any business owner but those who are further ahead. Those who are hungry. They know how to get to the next level and, in general, they like to turn around and help others level up, too.

Changing your inner circle can transform your business and your life.

I hope you found a great deal of value in this book. My goal was to provide as much practical advice and detail as possible while also keeping the book short enough so that people would actually read the entire thing. I know I never read those massive 2,000-page pharmacology textbooks cover to cover, did you?

With that said, if you find the possibility of opening your own clinic compelling and want more help in setting it up to be as successful as possible, I invite you to continue reading.

How to Know if You Need Help

You're not trying to open up a food cart here; you're trying to start a successful medical clinic. I can personally testify that operating a successful medical practice requires a completely different skill set and it will take time and effort to learn it. Don't be afraid to make mistakes. You will make them, I promise you. It's the nature of being human and pushing yourself. But mistakes can be super expensive.

One of the biggest mistakes you can make is *waiting to act*. People forget to factor opportunity cost into their business equation. Opportunity cost is the cost of the time and money you lose when you don't take the actions or, more importantly, when you don't take the *right* actions, needed to open your clinic.

You don't have to struggle to figure out how to open a clinic when other people who have done it can help and guide you through the process. You may think you are saving money by not investing in training programs, attorneys, accountants, or consultants, but the simple truth is, you're not.

You will pay dear for that decision in the amount of money you *could* have made and free time you could have had. Investing in a training program can shortcut your success and get you generating income much faster than trying to do it on your own.

Try this exercise: put a dollar amount on what your time is worth. Many healthcare professionals' time is worth a tremendous amount of money—often to the tune of hundreds of dollars per hour.

What if investing in a training program can save you dozens, if not hundreds, of hours? What if it prevented you from making tens of thousands of dollars in mistakes? If you think about it and do the math, investing in a training program led by other successful clinic owners is the only choice that makes any sense.

If you believe opening a cashed-based clinic could be your answer to a better life, greater impact, more freedom, and a better income, then I'd like to help you by inviting you to join one of my training programs.

When I started my clinic in 2017, programs like mine didn't exist, but boy, do I wish they had. That's why I spent the last five years building our programs, which include access to a private community of students *and* access to instructors and coaches, including myself.

The shift from W-2 employee to entrepreneur is a big one. A lot of what it takes is the right mindset; the rest is knowledge and grit. As a W-2 employee, other people dictate when you have to get up, when you have to drive to work, and what you do when you get there. They dictate how much time you get to spend with your friends and whether or not you get to eat a Thanksgiving meal with your family.

When you're an entrepreneur, you become a decision-maker, which is both awesome and kind of intimidating. You're not always going to know what you're doing or have the perfect information to choose a course of action. Entrepreneurship is all about making the best decisions you can with the information you have, moving forward, and then correcting your course if you get off track.

It takes an exceptional amount of initiative, and you have to be constantly learning and surrounding yourself with people who are smarter than you. Some people will resist that because they want to walk into a room and feel like they're the cream of the crop. Some like to stroke their egos by always feeling like they are the smartest person in the room. Believe me, a lot of healthcare professionals have huge egos. People with big egos make much better employees. It takes humility to build a business and to have a team to help build your practice.

If you are the type who can humble yourself and keep an open mind, you'll quickly find that when you hire and learn from people who are smarter than you or more experienced than you, your business will run better than you could even imagine.

Case in point … We have a Director of Operations who started as a virtual assistant (VA). Her name is Joyce, and she is a complete rockstar. She is a master of systems and processes, something I am weak at. She created a new hiring process for us including an entirely new applicant screening process.

Now, a person with a big—aka fragile—ego would feel threatened: "My VA is telling me how I should run my hiring process? Who do they think they are?" They'd probably ignore the person's ideas, assuming that their own ideas are better (what a jerk!). I didn't do that.

Joyce's idea for process improvement made our hiring process ten times better. Success takes collective effort which is something that is very unique about our training programs and mastermind. We have an amazing community of students and clinic owners who are collectively advising and assisting one another. They lift each other up and pull each other forward. It is amazing to see.

How Do You Find the Right Person to Help You? Ask Questions!

Have they accomplished what you want to accomplish?

There are some unethical clinic owners who are selling their consulting services—some have even sold franchises—all while never generating a dime of *profit* in their own practice. How do I know? Because I have had them reach out to me asking for help with their struggling clinics! So, buyer beware: seek out somebody who is, or has been, where you want to be. Don't ask just any business owner; ask a healthcare entrepreneur who started a profitable clinic. There are a lot of extra regulations and hurdles to overcome when you're in the healthcare space that most other entrepreneurs don't know anything about.

Most of the ethical experts you are going to find who fall into this category will charge for their services. After all, they could be growing their own business instead of helping others. Their time is valuable and frankly, they should charge for their expertise.

I know the first reaction might be to balk at spending the money. As we've said, the money you spend on having someone who knows what they're doing and coaches you will save you far more money and time in the long run. Wouldn't you rather pay a coach to be made aware of marketing strategies that are filling clinics up, rather than sitting alone in an empty office panicking because you have no clue how to attract revenue-generating patients?

Are their coaching or consulting clients successful?

A great coach has the ability to replicate success. They see where someone is falling short and know exactly the kind of help the person needs. When you're looking for someone who can possibly help, do your research. Look up past and present clients and see how their businesses are doing. Call them up and ask them about their experience and the results they have seen. We have an open Facebook group, and some of our members have shared horror stories about hiring consultants that charge ongoing royalties forever and provide no value for that recurring fee!

I highly recommend you talk to those clients. And let's get realistic here. 100% of people are not going to be successful, even with an amazing coach or consultant. Why? Because they fall into one of two categories:

1. They don't put in the work.
2. They aren't coachable.

If you avoid those pitfalls and find someone great to help you, your odds of success are very high. Success rate is not the only thing that matters though. What kind of person they are matters too.

Are they someone who builds their clients up, or do they tear them down?

Look at Steve Jobs. He's created one of the most profitable companies in history. But insiders have said that his idea of leadership was to berate and yell at people until they did what he wanted. Nowhere have we ever heard anyone say that he was a kind and patient teacher or mentor. His attitude and actions seriously affected his employees' quality of life. So, find help from someone who will support you, encourage you, and build you up.

Have they created a sellable business?

I've seen so many business owners, in both the medical field and outside of it, who have simply created another job for themselves. They still have to show up to their business day in and day out. If they want to take a vacation, they either have to close for the week or constantly check in to make sure everything is going well. Compare that to someone who has created systems and processes that allow their business to run whether they show up or not. You want a business where new patients are constantly coming in and for your staff to be able to handle every step of their treatment.

Do they provide direct support?

Are they available to help you? Will they walk you through your specific issues? Do they nickel and dime people or charge additional hourly consulting fees every time you have to ask a question? Find someone willing to provide you with the support you need to succeed and who is not going to upcharge you for every minute they spend helping you.

Being able to leverage the knowledge of people who know more than you is an advantageous strategy. Good mentors and coaches will lay out a roadmap for you that puts you light years ahead of others in your field. When someone is more knowledgeable than you, they help you see things from an eagle-eye view, and in that process, help you avoid stumbling blocks that they ran into during their own journey.

When you surround yourself with a community of people with whom you share similar interests, it is easy to find answers to questions and familiarize yourself with potential problems that arise in your field. You get ideas that you can key into, enhance, or customize to fit your situation.

Whether you are starting from scratch or already established, a little help, guidance, and collaboration go a long way toward getting you where you want to be. I've been there, so I can tell you first-hand how that goes. If you'd like to explore the possibility of working with me and our other instructors in one of our clinic training programs or mastermind, simply head on over to:

jasonduprat.com/book

Whether you choose to continue learning from and working with me or not, please know that it has been an honor to see you have made it to the end of this book. Please consider leaving a rating and review. I wish you the life of your dreams and success in whatever ventures you pursue. I will be rooting for you!

And remember, if you aren't where you want to be in life yet, you have a choice. It's your time to ...

"Stop Existing and Start Living."

—Jason A. Duprat

HOW TO ACCESS YOUR MIND-BLOWING BONUSES AND ADDITIONAL RESOURCES

Free MasterClasses with Start-Up Calculator Bonuses:

1. The Perfect Recipe for Starting a Successful IV Therapy Clinic

2. The 3 Proven Principles to Start and Grow a Profitable Ketamine Clinic

3. The 3 Secrets to Launching a Flourishing Med Spa

Ebooks:

1. *Boost Your Income with IV Therapy*

2. *Ketamine Business Jump Start*

3. *Med Spa Launch Made Easy*

Helpful Podcast Episodes:

#127 — "Dr. Vatsal Thakkar: Solving the Pain Point of Filing Claims with Reimbursify"

#233 — "Tom Wheelwright: Turning Income into Assets to Build Wealth"

#299 — "How to Find the Right Virtual Assistants for Your Medical Practice"

#303 — "Why It's Important to Optimize Your Clinic's Website for SEO"

#304 — "Tactical Tuesday: How to Earn Positive ROI from Joining a Mastermind Event"

#305 — "Sales, Marketing, and Rapport-Building: How to Avoid Common Mistakes and Misconceptions"

To learn more about our **Exclusive Clinic Growth Expert Mastermind** and access your **FREE bonuses and ebooks**—as well as **hundreds more podcast episodes**—go here:

jasonduprat.com/book

STUDENT AND
CLIENT TESTIMONIALS

Jason A. Duprat and his team have given me all the tools organized by topic which has saved me many hours and headaches. As if all this were not enough, there is a "Bonuses" section with the necessary documentation that with a couple of clicks, I adapted to my business. Another great strength is the exclusive Facebook group where there are other entrepreneurs who are in the same process and who ask and answer questions that appear on a daily basis during the creation of the business. I honestly believe that the value well outweighs the price. Thank you all!

—Miguel S. Porto, MD

Despite practicing Emergency Medicine as a Board Certified physician, I was reluctant to make the leap into private practice. Jason's course was clear and concise and helped me focus on what was needed to open my clinic within months of completing the course. Small important nuances left out of other courses were made easy to understand and reaffirmed what I knew already. This was something I could do, help people, and have a renewed sense of freedom. I'm able to actually practice the art of medicine once again, on my own terms. My first month open, I was overwhelmed with calls and completed 15 infusions with text messages like, "Thank you for fixing my brain, Dr. Pellegrino. No more anxiety!" So, thank you, Jason, for helping me regain my freedom.

—Michael Pellegrino, DO

This is the course to take if you have wondered how in the heck you will know if you've covered everything before you open your own clinic. This course takes you from step one, which explains why you should open a clinic. The best part of the entire course is Jason provides the forms and literature already. You have to do minimal research. Jason does it all. You can't beat the price when everything is included. Not only that, you can get pre-approved CEUs from the AANA. What a deal!

—Kathy Burgess, APRN, CRNA

I was in a place where I wanted to be my own boss. I wanted to spend more time with my child and my family. I was tired of working 40, 50, 60 hours a week. So I looked into Jason Duprat's IV Therapy Academy. I had no idea about IV hydration. Now I know it's just such a wonderful, beneficial thing for all walks of life. It was kind of scary because I don't know anything about having a business. The course literally walks you through everything. I'm glad I had this course.

—Amanda Eagan, DNP, CRNA

I'm sitting in my office, Wholistic Health. Without Ketamine Academy, I would not be here. I wouldn't have my own clinic. Ketamine Academy really gives you all the tools that you need, which is fabulous. You understand how ketamine works, the efficacy of ketamine, how to build your business, and advertising. It is fantastic. I have to tell you, I refer back to the coursework all the time. The Facebook page is invaluable to help in figuring everything out. Jason's a great support person to help you do this. You can start your own clinic, and you can have a good clinic. Jason's course is AMAZING. Please take it. I recommend his course to all my friends. It really does give you everything you need.

—Susan Gillispie, APRN

Excellent, very helpful, and provided exactly what I needed as an MD who has never run his own clinic. Very practical advice all the way down to where to get good deals on equipment and supplies, how to process payments, issues with scope of practice, insurance, and building leases. Thank you so much for helping me to start out right and avoid making a myriad of mistakes.

—Eric Milbrandt, MD

I always wanted to run an IV clinic. I think it is very helpful to so many people to improve their quality of life. Because I didn't know too much about laws, regulations, and policies, it has been a challenge. This course has helped me learn more about policies and how to avoid mistakes. My favorite thing about this course is I think everyone is very dedicated. I have learned so much about running a clinic, the cost, policies, supplies, and pharmacy regulations. This course is amazing!

—Cuicui Zhang, APRN

I thoroughly recommend this course to anyone who is thinking about starting up their own practice. Basically, in less than 2.5 months, I've been able to go from ZERO knowledge of how to start a practice to a pretty good understanding of everything that I need and everything that I have to put in place prior to being able to practice. This is completely because of the Ketamine Academy and Jason.

—Bobby Hill, APRN

Jason is there to help and get you through with your questions. Jason's course is very thorough and informative. If you are not sure whether to take the course or not, it is definitely worth your while.

—Charlie Hong, CRNA

I want to give credit to Jason's thoroughness and level of attention to detail. Well worth the investment!

—Jon Wolfe, EMT-P

Jason's course takes you through everything you need to know, clinical and business to get your own clinic up and running.

—Dana Cochrane-Hoekstra, PA

I believe one of the most important aspects of running a successful practice is to stay consistent and compliant. Practicing safety and delivering transparency are guidelines that we should all follow. The IV Therapy Academy has set these guidelines and knowledge to efficiently prepare you to have a successful practice. I highly recommend IV Therapy Academy to all who want to start IV Hydration therapies the right way while practicing safely with your clients.

—Leslie V.M., APRN

Ketamine Academy was instrumental in helping me get my clinic up and going quickly and efficiently. I strongly recommend Ketamine Academy to anyone who is wanting to open up their own clinic or their own business. It will definitely save you a lot of time and money in getting yourself started.

—Tyler Thornock, CRNA

I'm so glad I stumbled upon IV Therapy Academy. I struggled with knowing how to start establishing an LLC, I didn't know who to talk to, and I didn't know who the professionals were that I needed in my corner. Jason and KC have been so supportive along the way!

—Madeline Price, BSN, RN, FNP-C

Jason is always there, every step of the way. There hasn't been one point where I have not gotten a great answer to a question. Without him, I could have never done this. I can never thank Jason enough for the schedule and income freedom to enjoy my kids and husband more than I ever imagined! I appreciate you, Jason, for your knowledge, patience, and continued mentorship as I evolve strategies to help CRNAs "leap" to a better life! With your online educational program and mentorship, you have certainly helped me achieve a wonderfully free lifestyle! I applaud your success!

—Alesia Quante, MHSA, CRNA

WHAT IS A HEALTHCARE BOSS?

*"A tribe is a group of people who are connected to one
another, to their community, and to their culture. It's a place
where you belong and feel a sense of connection and support."*

—Seth Godin

The Healthcare Boss is a new breed of healthcare professional ...

We are nurses, doctors, and other healthcare professionals who
realize that our healthcare system is broken *and* is reaching a
point of no return.

It is now a system controlled by investors and administrators who seek
to maximize profits at the expense of their workers and their patients.

Healthcare Bosses are passionate professionals who deeply care
for their patients and believe that patients always come first.

A Healthcare Boss knows that working for corporate medicine is
no longer the only way, nor does corporate medicine have them
or their patients' best interests in mind.

As Healthcare Boss clinicians we want to care for patients on our
terms, and we want to regain our freedom and autonomy. We
know there is a better way.

We are healthcare professionals who choose to earn an independent living by:

1. Practicing in a way we're proud of,
2. Providing services focused on the health and wellness of patients,
3. Offering treatments and services worth paying for.

The Healthcare Boss sees what's broken in corporate medicine and finds solutions that matter to the patients we aim to serve.

We abhor the current model of disease management and assembly-line healthcare.

We know the dirty healthcare secret—corporate medicine, big pharma, and insurance companies all put profits ahead of people.

Healthcare Bosses create patient-focused businesses that improve the lives of others, allowing us to earn a respectable income without having to sacrifice the most important aspects of our lives.

This allows the healthcare boss to serve first, but do it on their own time and in their own way so they don't succumb to burnout and exhaustion.

We truly believe that we *do not* need to give up our entire lives in service to Corporate Medicine.

For us, creating an independent living with our own businesses means complete control and freedom of how we practice and how we serve. We are excited about the work we do!

It means freedom to solve the problems that we find interesting and are for the betterment of patients ... so we feel good about our contributions.

That's the formula for happiness right there.

If you see yourself as someone who wants to change the healthcare industry (on a big or small scale) by serving patients and clients on your terms, you're in the right place.

Welcome to our Tribe.

We aim to help healthcare professionals create their own healthcare businesses that are free from the red tape and greed of corporate medicine and third-party payors.

Businesses and private practices that allow us the freedom to earn a good living while still being home for dinner, holidays, and the other important moments that have been taken from us.

The formula is simple, but is it not always easy:

1. Find a group of patients or businesses with a problem they need to solve,

2. Align it with a solution you're excited to deliver and make it so good they're excited to pay for it!

3. Create happy patients or clients. Serve patients in a way that makes them eager to lead a better, healthier life. And serve your clients in a way that helps their operation run smoothly and they will tell everyone that you were the one who helped them achieve the outcome!

The Healthcare Boss makes their patients and clients feel like they matter because they do!

Most healthcare professionals are stuck in an old and outdated dogma … Believing that 10 minutes and a few questions will tell them what they need to know in order to prescribe the next pill (usually to cover up symptoms of the last pill) and they never stop to think that more pills might not be the best answer.

Big Pharma and Corporate Medicine have taken over our education and taught us that anything outside of their doctrine is heresy and voodoo magic, unfit even to have a conversation about. Their only goal is to maintain the status quo and continue to pad the pockets of those at the top.

No thanks.

That's not us.

The Healthcare Boss practicing clinically believes that the only way to serve our patients is to explore all options, look at everything, and have hard conversations. To ask questions like:

- "Does this really work?"
- "Is this what's best for my patient?"
- "Am I addressing the root cause of the problem?"

And they have the courage to change course if the answer is no.

This is why the Healthcare Boss believes in independent practices and other business models that allow for maximum control. It gives them the freedom to practice in a way that best serves their patients while allowing them the autonomy to pivot when new evidence is presented.

The Healthcare Boss isn't stuck in old dogma simply because "this is how we've always done it." They're on the cutting edge, keeping up with new research while taking a critical look at the quality and truth of that research.

This allows them to serve patients and provide services that others are happy to pay for.

Our Mission: To serve our patients and clients first, in a way that truly matters to them. To help others and do it in a way that supports our own independence and freedom.

If you have a desire to serve first, in a way that matters, then we think you'll love what we have in store for you.

Our Healthcare Entrepreneur Academy has helped thousands become #HealthcareBosses through teaching others how to break free from corporate medicine by starting their own businesses.

But that's only the beginning.

Now it's time to start a revolution by creating more Healthcare Bosses who are ready and willing to serve others in a way that truly matters, all while expanding their personal and professional freedom.

Thank you for joining the revolution and allowing us to serve you along your entrepreneurial journey.

We are excited and know the future holds some amazing possibilities for you.

The question is: *Will you step out of your comfort zone and start taking action?*

Only you know the answer, but just know we are here to support you when you are ready to take that leap of faith …

ACKNOWLEDGMENTS

I want to thank my parents, Humberto and Melinda, you instilled the values, faith, and work ethic that have propelled me through life. Thank you for always keeping me pointed in the right direction. Even if I didn't seem to appreciate it, I did.

To my middle school teacher, Mrs. Pat Will, when many others saw nothing more than a decent wrestler in me, you saw far more. I will never know what you noticed back then, but you relentlessly challenged me and built me up—and because of this, I am here today. Cheers to saying "I told you so" to all the naysayers!

Thanks to all the amazing entrepreneurs I have learned from who have helped me create businesses that allow me to wake up excited nearly every day. Businesses that helped me escape my prison cell of a call room, along with some of the darkest days of my professional life. Businesses that put me back in the driver's seat, in complete control of my personal and professional destiny. Without the inspiration and motivation I gained from you, I would certainly still be sitting in my comfort zone, punching that time clock, and counting down the hours until my next day off.

John Lee Dumas, your podcast, *Entrepreneurs On Fire*, was my saving grace. Listening to hundreds of your episodes helped me realize that I could do it; I could start my own business. After about a year of listening, I started my own clinic and shortly after, my first academy.

A huge thanks to both you *and* Kate Erickson for hosting the mastermind at your beautiful home in Puerto Rico. That was my first-ever mastermind, and it was a life-changing event. You analyzed my new business along with my financial situation and gave me the confidence I needed to quit my anesthesia job so that I could go all-in as an entrepreneur. JLD I still have the picture of "QUIT" written by you in giant red letters when you told me what you believed I needed to do next. Thanks to both of you, I quit my job before the mastermind was even finished. It was one of the best decisions of my life!

I want to thank Travis Chappell, founder of Guestio and creator of the *Build Your Network* podcast, now called *Travis Makes Friends*. Your coaching and mentorship gave me the tools to create one of the top-rated healthcare business podcasts. Thanks for all the supportive phone calls and great tips, from how to launch all the way to getting top-tier podcast guests. Without your help and guidance, my podcast wouldn't even exist.

I want to thank all our 4,000+ students. You entrusted me to guide you through your entrepreneurial journey, and that is an honor I don't take lightly. An extra special thank you goes out to all my die-hard, go-getter students who put in the work, methodically attended dozens of our coaching calls and took the action needed to launch their businesses successfully. I have probably learned more from you than I have from spending hundreds of hours researching. Nothing energizes me more than to work with a group of hungry, ambitious, and smart professionals like yourselves. You are the backbone that has created our tribe of healthcare bosses; thank you for passing it forward by helping the newest members of our courses and community. Hats off to you all.

Thank you to our entire team, especially our Director of Operations, Joyce P. You are all amazing at filling in the gaps, covering for my weaknesses, and taking outstanding care of our customers. Thank you for putting up with my incessant tendencies to try to oversee every detail and for having the courage to tell me when you've got it; also for some killer ideas and suggestions. It was the strength of our team that allowed me to "go dark" for weeks to finish this book. Lastly, thanks for sticking with me when we made the difficult transition from running the business part-time, like a hobby, to running it like a real company. I know that wasn't easy; we lost a few along the way, but thankfully, you all made it to the other side. I look forward to many more years together.

I would like to express my deepest gratitude to Shanda Trofe of Transcendent Publishing and our editor Lori Lynn for their invaluable support and guidance throughout the writing and publishing process of this book. Their expertise and commitment to excellence have been instrumental in bringing this project to fruition. Thank you for your dedication and hard work.

Most importantly, thank you, the reader. Thank you for investing in this book and for taking the time to read it. If nothing else, I hope this book opens your eyes to all the incredible business opportunities that are out there waiting for you. This is just the first step to grabbing the reins and forging a new path that can allow you to live the personal and professional life of your dreams.

ABOUT THE AUTHOR

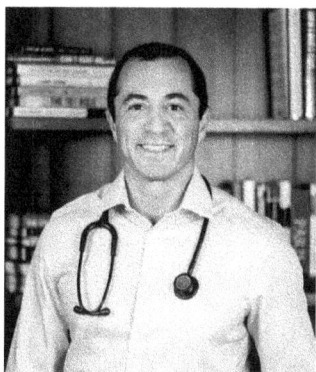

Jason A. Duprat is a serial entrepreneur, nurse anesthetist, and former nurse corps naval officer of nearly 10 years. During his first 11 years working in the corporate healthcare system, he began to gain an insider's perspective on how the US healthcare system actually works.

After years of increasing burnout, Jason decided to forge his own path by starting a successful clinic. Practitioners from around the country took notice and sought him out to help them escape the corporate grind through practice ownership. He loved helping other clinicians so much that he founded the Healthcare Entrepreneur Academy, IV Therapy Academy, Med Spa Launch Academy, and Ketamine Academy.

Jason is also the creator of the *Healthcare Entrepreneur Academy* podcast where he has published over 310 episodes and interviewed over 140 healthcare entrepreneurs and other business experts.

Jason believes business ownership is the key to a happy and fulfilling career as a professional in today's healthcare environment. Through his training programs, Jason has helped thousands of healthcare professionals.

To connect with or learn more about Jason, follow him on LinkedIn at **linkedin.com/in/jasonaduprat/** or head over to **JasonDuprat.com**.

www.ingramcontent.com/pod-product-compliance
Lightning Source LLC
Chambersburg PA
CBHW070657190326
41458CB00053B/6918/J